IN SEARCH OF
THE FOUNTAIN OF YOUTH

C. C. HARRELL, NCC, MS, RN

FIRST EDITION

THE HEALTH FORUM PUBLISHING COMPANY
Memphis, Tennessee 38101-9715

HEALTH 卄 FORUM

The Health Forum Publishing Company
P.O. Box 844
Memphis, Tennessee 38101-9715

Library of Congress Catalog Card Number: 91-071017

ISBN 0-9629247-0-9

Printed in the United States of America

Additional copies may be ordered from:
Cindy Harrell
Health Forum Publishing Company
P.O. Box 844
Memphis, Tennessee, 38101-9715

DEDICATION

This book is primarily dedicated to THE **GODHEAD (THE FATHER, SON, AND THE HOLY SPIRIT), Creator of the heaven and the earth.**

Secondly, it is dedicated to those individuals who are mentally, physically, spiritually, or situationally handicapped (especially the homeless).

Thirdly, it is dedicated to the precious memory of my parents, the late Mr. Cleveland and Mrs. Rosie Clayton.

Fourthly, it is dedicated to my son and daughter-in-law, James & Cindy Harrell; and to my two grandsons, James E. Harrell, III and Cidny Harrell.

ACKNOWLEDGEMENTS

T HANK You Dear God, Creator of the heaven and the earth, for using me to be Your human instrument to present this message.

Your most gracious, humble, and loyal servant,

C. C. Harrell

A special thanks to my son and daughter-in-law, James and Cindy Harrell. Without your prayers, words of encouragement, and physical labor, this book would still be in the very early stages of development.

Also, thanks to my many friends, relatives, and co-workers for their prayers and words of encouragement.

The cover and all graphics were developed by Cindy Harrell under **specific** guidance of the Holy Spirit. We all thank the WordPerfect Corporation for giving her permission to use their software program to produce the cover and graphics.

CONTENTS

Section I.

SEARCHING FOR A FOUNTAIN

Section II.

THE FOUNTAIN LOCATED

Section III.

Resuming Our Journey: This Time In Search of The Basic Principles of Health

Section IV.

Everyday Problems Find Solutions Through God's Commandments, Laws, Statues, and Principles

Section V.

THE GREATEST GIFT

APPENDIX, REFERENCES, and INDEX

PREFACE

WHEN one listens to the concerns that are plaguing the American society today, it is noted that the same topics surface over and over. Such topics are: _SUBSTANCE ABUSE_, _CRIME_, _TEEN PREGNANCIES_, _POOR HEALTH_, _THE HIGH COSTS OF HEALTH SERVICES_, _OBESITY_, _EXCESSIVE STRESS_, _AND SEARCHING FOR METHODS TO INCREASE THE QUALITY AND QUANTITY OF LIFE_.

There is a tremendous amount of confusion about which factors really impact health. This confusion has resulted in appalling statistics in this country as far as health indicators are concerned.   Sickness and other problems have become accepted as "status quo" and inevitable.

Fortunately, there are those of us in our society who are not satisfied with the "status quo". We are ready to take a journey to _**SEARCH**_ for serious answers to some of these problems.

All of the concerns are of equal importance; and if there were sufficient time and energy, we would search for the answers to all of them. Of course, it is unlikely that we will be able to search for **ALL** of the answers to **ALL** of the problems on one journey, so we must carefully select the target of our exploration.

The words "**sufficient time and energy**" can be looked upon as the key words to help us mark the course of our journey. We will conduct this search by looking for the methods which increase the **QUALITY and QUANTITY of LIFE.** Perhaps, if we find these answers, they will give us the time and energy to search through some of the other concerns.

Typically, anything that is capable of increasing the QUALITY and QUANTITY of life is referred to as a **FOUNTAIN OF YOUTH.** In essence, we are going to **SEARCH FOR THE FOUNTAIN OF YOUTH.**

INTRODUCTION

W E are not the first to search for THE FOUNTAIN OF YOUTH in an effort to increase the quality and quantity of life. On March 3, 1513, Ponce de Leon, a Spanish Explorer, set sail from San German, Puerto Rico. Legend had it that he was searching for the Land of Bimini. This land was believed to contain a **"FOUNTAIN"** with "curative powers". The fountain, now referred to as the **FOUNTAIN OF YOUTH,** spurted forth a rejuvenating tonic spring which caused all who drank from it or bathed in it to be cured from diseases and live a long, healthy life.

On April 2, 1513, Ponce de Leon landed in what is now known as Florida. Although originally, he had no intention of landing there; nevertheless, Florida became associated with the legend of the **FOUNTAIN OF YOUTH.** Later the **FOUNTAIN OF YOUTH** became associated with America in general.

There is no documented evidence that Ponce de Leon ever found the fountain that he sought. But, at the same time, equally true is the fact that there is no definite proof that such a fountain does _NOT_ exist.

Let us just stop and imagine for a moment--a real **FOUNTAIN OF YOUTH,** spurting forth a tangible elixir or some type of liquid which is capable of curing diseases and positively influencing longevity. If we could find the key to unlock such a miraculous secret, imagine the possibilities: freedom from diseases, longevity, peace, tranquility, ad infinitum.

As we ponder over the issue, we note that, if we were to find such a fountain, why settle for just a long healthy life? Why not check out the possibility of **LIVING FOREVER** and never having to worry about death or illness again? Just think, never having to say goodbye to friends and loved ones. Just thinking about this makes us all excited and tingly inside.

But, of course, in modern times we acknowledge the fact there is no such thing as a **FOUNTAIN OF YOUTH -- OR -- IS THERE?** Since there is no specific proof that the **FOUNTAIN OF YOUTH** does _NOT_ exist, maybe it would be a worthwhile venture to check into this matter for ourselves. Just as Ponce de Leon searched, we too can begin a journey _IN SEARCH OF THE FOUNTAIN OF YOUTH....._

STARTING THE SEARCH

To begin our search, we could get on a boat and sail the seas as did Ponce de Leon. Or, we could hop a plane or grab a bus or train. But, just as with our Spanish explorer of yesteryear, a search of this type could prove costly, time consuming, and fruitless. Since we are already limited by time, energy, finance, and even intellect; it is reasonable that we conduct our voyage in a different way. Our unique method of searching could save time, energy, money, and even enhance our intellect to a certain degree. Our voyage, of course, will maneuver us through the encyclopedias, medical journals, dictionaries, and other books of the library. As we travel, we are desperately searching for a hint or clue that will lead us to our destination; *IN SEARCH OF THE FOUNTAIN OF YOUTH!*

IN Sᴇᴀʀᴄʜ *OF*

Tʜᴇ Fᴏᴜɴᴛᴀɪɴ Oғ Yᴏᴜᴛʜ

Section I.

SEARCHING FOR A FOUNTAIN

LEG 1

BEGINNING OUR JOURNEY

WE are going to conduct this search in a manner similar to that of a detective searching for clues in a very special case. A good detective would begin the search by learning as much as possible about the subject itself. So, the first leg of our journey will, logically, begin with finding a good definition of the term "fountain" and then reaching mutuality on the aspect of "youth" that we seek. With this task completed, we will have a specific understanding of that which we seek.

Funk and Wagnall's Standard College Dictionary defines the word "fountain" as follows:

- a spring or jet of liquid issuing from the earth.

- the source of a stream.

- the origin or source of anything.

- a jet spray of liquid forced upward.

The Academic American Encyclopedia, Volume 8, page 251 informs us that "fountains" are channels or sprouts through which water is directed under pressure.

The Encyclopedia American, Volume II, page 1650 speaks of water being forced, by pressure, through pipes, conduits, or aqueducts.

Pipes are familiar to us, but not "aqueducts" and "conduits". Perhaps we should do a little exploration on these two terms before we can determine the exact direction of our search.

So, back to Funk and Wagnall's. We see such words as "acquaint, aquavit, aquavitae". Oh, here we are "aqueduct". An aqueduct is defined as:

- a water conduit, especially one for supplying water to a community from a distance.

- any of several canals through which *BODY FLUIDS* are conducted.

Webster defines an aqueduct as "a course, channel, or bridge for covering water; either under or above the ground".

The word "conduit" is basically synonymous with "aqueduct". It is defined as a covered passage or tube. Now, what do we know or wish to know about the term "youth"? As we search through the various dictionaries, we find such definitions as:

■ the state or quality of being young.

■ the state of being vigorous and lively.

■ fresh, active.

■ an early stage of growth or existence.

■ the period of life between childhood and maturity.

■ immature, impetuous.

Our reason tells us that once we are born into the world there is nothing that will influence the chronological aging process. So we know that this fountain that we are seeking won't make us sixteen again, nor twenty-five for that matter. We definitely have no desire for immaturity or impetuousness which are the inevitable companions of youth.

Through the process of elimination, we choose the statements which deal with being fresh, lively, vigorous, and active from our definitions of youth listed above. These two statements identify some of the benefits that we hope to reap from this great elixir spurting forth from the *FOUNTAIN OF YOUTH.*

So, we are looking for an elixir to increase vigor, liveliness, and activity. And, of course, it will also need to possess the capability to render us free from diseases and may even be a factor in causing us to live forever.

SUMMARIZING THE DIMENSIONS OF THE SEARCH

The first leg of our journey has provided us with a reasonable idea of what we are searching for. So, let's summarize the information that we have gathered thus far and put it into the proper perspective. The factors listed below provide the basic information related to this very special elixir that we are searching for on our journey *IN SEARCH OF THE FOUNTAIN OF YOUTH.* This very special elixir is:

■   a substance which is a liquid. No, we are not searching for water. True, water is totally essential for life, but as we will see, all of the factors listed do not apply to water.

■   a substance which is in constant motion.

■   constantly moving under pressure through something similar to pipes, conduits, and aqueducts. This fact allows us to conclude that under normal circumstances this substance is covered.

■ possibly, even some type of body fluid.

■ capable of giving us the feeling, appearance, and reality of being vigorous, lively, fresh, and active, and of course, rendering us free from diseases. Also, it may cause us to live forever.

There is a major question concerning this miraculous elixir. *IS IT REALLY POSSIBLE THAT IT CAN CAUSE US TO LIVE FOREVER?* We'll just have to answer that question when we find the fountain.

So, we pack these few clues in our bags and begin a serious journey *IN SEARCH OF THE FOUNTAIN OF YOUTH.*

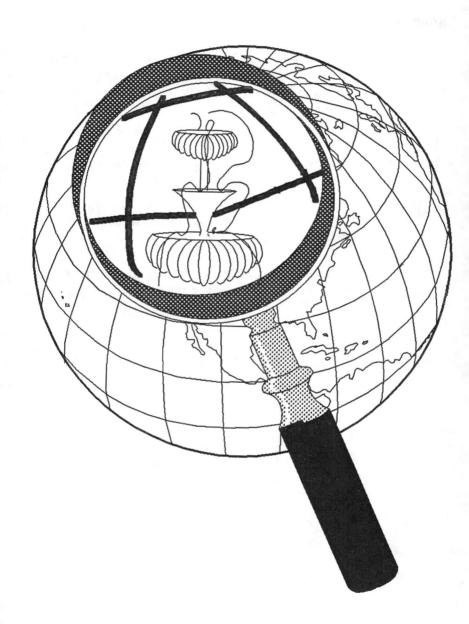

LEG 2

A CLOSER LOOK AT THE FOUNTAINS OF THE WORLD

S INCE we are *IN SEARCH OF A FOUNTAIN;* logically, we will take a look at some of the well-known fountains of the world. Perhaps it is here that we will reach our destiny and locate the *Fountain of Youth.*

As we maneuver through the mountains of papers, books, journals, and encyclopedias, we learn a lot of interesting information about fountains.

The earliest fountains date back to ancient Babylon and Greece (4000 B.C.). Originally, they were all natural but man has learned to manipulate and harness water to move in various directions for decorative, drinking, or irrigation purposes.

As we veer through this leg of our search, we move from Ancient Babylon and Greece to Italy where we see the elaborate gardens of the Emperor Hardrian in the Palace at Tivoli (these fountains were constructed between A.D. 118 & A.D. 134). Our minds sail through Giovanni da Bologna's Neptune Fountain (constructed between 1563 - 1567), Giovanni Lorenzo Berninis Fountain of the Four Rivers (1648 - 1659), and Nicola Salvi's Trevi Fountain (1732 - 1762).

With excitement, we explore fountains of the 20th century. We note Alexander Calder's *Water Ballet* at General Motors Company Building in Detroit, Michigan (constructed in 1954); the IBM Headquarters in Armonk, New York (built in 1964) by Isamu Noguchi; Carl Milles' Fountain, The Meeting Place (constructed in 1940) in St. Louis, Missouri; and Charles Moore's St. Joseph's Fountain in the Pizza d'Italia (constructed in 1978).

We pause for a minute to recap and evaluate all of the things that we have learned. We have picked up a lot of information, but sadly, we are no closer to the location of the *Fountain of Youth* than when we first began.

Though disappointed, we are not defeated--no--not this early in the game. We vow to leave no stone unturned. There are many other areas for us to explore. We anxiously move to the next leg of our journey, still *IN SEARCH OF THE FOUNTAIN OF YOUTH.*

LEG 3

EXPLORING ARCHITECTURE:
THE MOST USEFUL OF ALL ARTS

W E stand steadfast in our vow to leave no stone unturned. As we ponder over which field to next search, these interesting facts come to our attention about architecture. Architecture is defined as the art of erecting structures and is noted to be the most useful of all the fine arts. Surely, we will find some helpful hints or clues here.

As we wade through the information available, we learn that the most ancient Egyptian structures were built between 2686 & 248 B. C. We marvel as we peer at the sphinxes and lions.

11

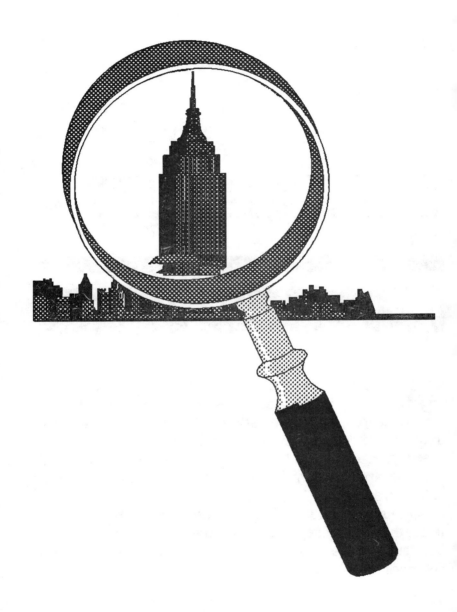

We soon change focus and soar through the architectural structures of the Babylonian (1900 - 1500 B.C.) and the Assyrian Empires (1100 - 612 B.C.). We note the massive brick platforms raised above the flood plain. We visually partake of the further ziggurated form. We learn that the Persian Empire (538 - 333 B.C.) adopted these features and supplemented them with the extensive use of columns, as in the palaces of Persepolis (516 - 460 B.C.).

We glide through Greece and become aware of The Great Minoan Palaces on the Island of Crete. In particular, we note the huge complex of Knossos and the magnificently sited structures at Phaistos. These masterpieces were constructed between 1700 and 1400 B.C.

After the Greeks developed the vocabulary of architecture, this vocabulary became fundamental to European architecture for more than 2,000 years.

While wandering through Rome we learn that the most significant achievement of the Romans was in the "technology" of building. They used a much wider range of materials and refined the Vault and the Dome. They built Aqueducts, Thermae such as the Baths of Caracalla, Basilicas (law courts), theaters, triumphal arches, amphitheaters, and palaces which involved enclosing much larger spaces, and of bridging much greater distances than could be achieved by using the standard timbers or stone beams. As we continue on our journey through Roman architecture, we learn about the Pantheon in Rome (a domed structure erected 120 - 123 A.D.). We peer at the Ravenna (534 - 539 A.D.) and the Huge Dome Church Hagia Sophia (532 - 537 A.D.).

We pick up such tidbits as, "from the mid 12th century to the 16th century, the Northern European Arch was characterized by the use of flying buttresses pointed arches, ribbed vaults, and traceried windows". All that we have encountered make us feel well-informed. We have soared through the field of architecture, the most useful of the fine arts. It has been informative and interesting. Beneficial in our search?; no, not in the least. So we leave the field of architecture with no more clues than when we started. The "most useful of the fine arts" has not been useful to us in our journey. But we are still *IN SEARCH OF THE FOUNTAIN OF YOUTH.*

LEG 4

ENGINEERING: A REASONABLE PLACE TO SEARCH

WELL, now into which direction shall we MOVE? There are still many areas from which to choose. We must select our road logically. The field of engineering looks perfect. It is the profession which deals with the design and building of machines, devices, and structures. We are told that though it is a very old profession, it has been only in the eighteenth century that the engineer has been distinguished from the scientist, the inventor, and the builder. In ancient times the term engineering applied to the building of irrigation canals,

15

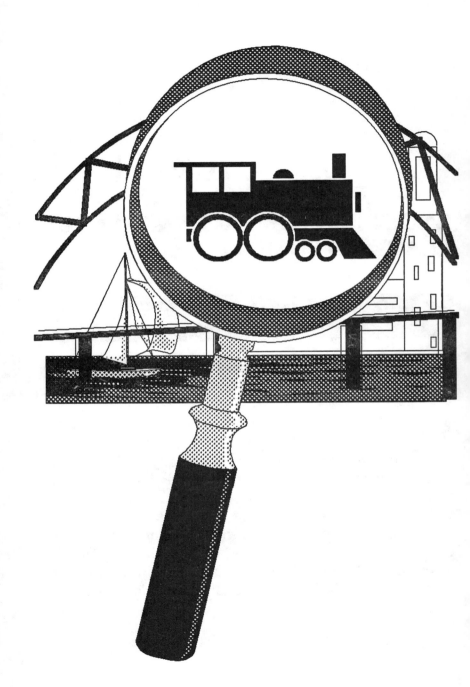

dams, palaces, temples, roads, and other facilities to satisfy the needs of mankind. Look at this statement, "Engineering involves a body of knowledge of mathematical and natural sciences gained by study, experience, and practice applied with judgement to develop ways to economically utilize the materials and forces of nature for the benefit of mankind." This definition, written by the Engineers Council for Professional Development, was found in the Academic Encyclopedia Vol. _7_.

Further reading related to the field of engineering informs us that before designs of certain structures could be made, it was necessary to develop certain tools. As we search through the literature, we read about the lathe and building materials such as: the various metals, cementing materials, concrete, building stones, clay products, insulating materials, bituminous materials, timber, and light-weight, high-quality steel.

After wading through the branches of engineering: aeronautical, agricultural, bioengineering, ceramics, chemical, civil, electrical, and industrial; we continue our search by moving through terms pertaining to engineering such as ductility, hardness, resistance, plasticity, and malleability. We almost strain our brains to understand the various tests that the materials must go through: tensile test, compressive-strength test, flexural strength test, hardness testing, impact test, creep test, corrosion test, and the fatigue test. WE ARE NOW FATIGUED.

Once again we have learned a lot of interesting facts; still, we have not one helpful clue. So, we must look elsewhere *IN SEARCH OF THE FOUNTAIN OF YOUTH.*

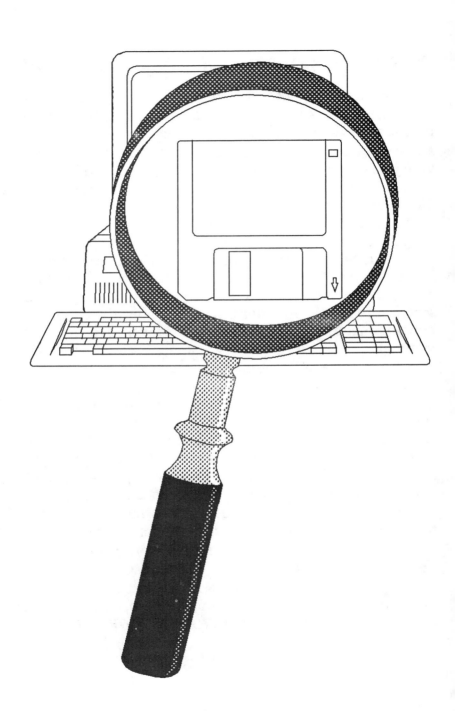

LEG 5

TECHNOLOGY: WHY NOT?

W E have not yet become weary in our quest for *THE FOUNTAIN OF YOUTH*. Nevertheless, in order to remain enthused, we must go back and review our vow to leave no stone unturned. Now we are aware of the benefits of traveling through the library rather than through actual locations. If we were traveling in the routine manner, we would have long since run out of time, money, energy, and patience.

The field of technology is the field that we have chosen to next search. It is defined as the application of science and technical advances in industry, manufacturing, commerce, and art. French Sociologist, Jacques Ellul defined it as "the totality of all national methods in every field of human activity". Technology has had a major impact on human lives and is said to be no less important in shaping human culture than philosophy, religion, social organization, or political systems.

The history of technology began with the use of stone tools by the earliest humans and has led us to modern-time inventions like complex computers. We sail through the Bronze age, the Iron age, the Roman and Medieval periods, the Renaissance, and the 18th, 19th, and 20th centuries. We are truly amazed at the advancements in every area of industry and art. We move from the radio to television and to video cassette recorders. We hop from the phonograph to audio tapes. We blaze through a trail wide enough to cover everything from the washing machine to modern-day rockets and computers. We even take a glance at the super computers.

We marvel at such information as:

■   Computers, though not as elaborate and efficient as they are today, existed since the 17th century.

■   In 1887 the German Physicist, Heinrich Hertz discovered that he could use sparks to produce radio waves by purely electrical means. He used a simple receiver to pick up waves fifty feet away.

We must admit to being fascinated and amused. This line of study could go on much longer, but, we can't get carried away. We must remember the purpose of our journey. Once again we have picked up a lot of interesting facts, but we are no closer to our goal than at the start of our journey. So as we leave the field of technology, we ponder over the path that we will next tread *IN SEARCH OF THE FOUNTAIN OF YOUTH.*

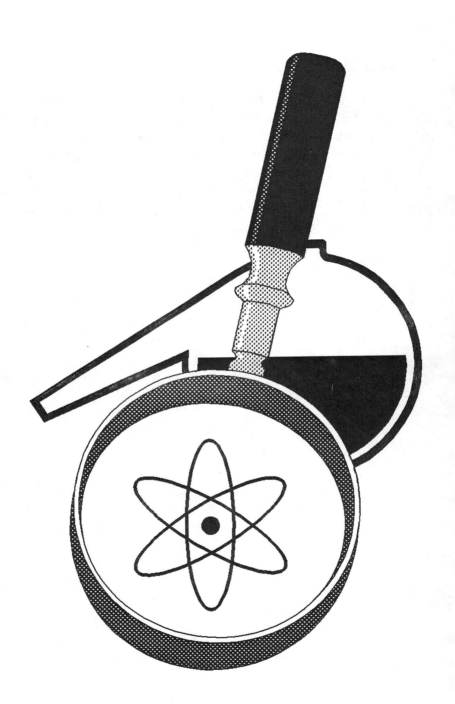

LEG 6

SCIENCE: A LIKELY PLACE TO SEARCH

"SCIENCE out shines everything since the rise of Christianity." This statement was made by scientist, Herbert Butterfield. In other text, science is described as a field of study arising from the need to make sense of the world through observation and investigation.

We certainly want to "make sense of the world"; so, we choose this field as the next area to explore on our journey. We make stops along the way to check out the accomplishments of Aristotle, Isaac Newton, Francis Bacon,

Madame Currie, and Aguste Comte. We peer and probe as we observe information about Stevenson's rocket and the space crafts of today. We move back to the discovery of the electric battery in the eighteen hundreds. We also take a look at Rutherford's work on the atom and we take time to check out nuclear fission.

We are impressed to learn that scientific advancements walked hand-in-hand with truth and progress for two centuries. It is with great concern and even grief that as we surge through the pages of the encyclopedias, we find that since the 1970s, scientific research has become the subject of much debate and mistrust. There are statements about secret research and information that has been withheld.

Once again we have searched an interesting field; but we have found no truly useful information that will help us on our journey *IN SEARCH OF THE FOUNTAIN OF YOUTH.*

LEG 7

A UNIQUE SEARCH THROUGH THE STATUS OF AMERICAN HEALTH

W E have searched through mountains of literature which told us of fountains, architecture, engineering, technology, and science. Yet, we are no closer to finding clues related to the location of the *FOUNTAIN OF YOUTH* than when we first began. We made a vow to leave no stone unturned. So, we move on. Once again we ponder over the path that we shall next tread. We are beginning to feel perplexed. But, we still believe that a *FOUNTAIN OF YOUTH* does exist. We even begin to research our own notes from the beginning of this journey. In the Introduction (page xvi), we made the point that

STATUS _____ H

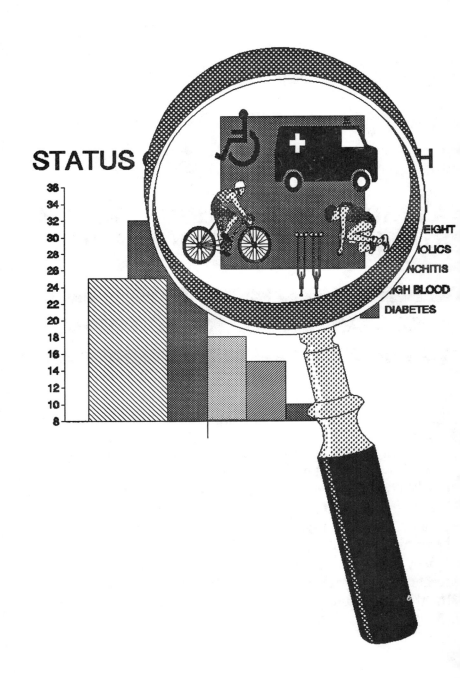

EIGHT
OLICS
NCHITIS
GH BLOOD
DIABETES

36
34
32
30
28
26
24
22
20
18
16
14
12
10
8

America is associated with *The Fountain of Youth;* and on page 6, we noted that *The Fountain of Youth* is associated with freedom from disease. Freedom from disease means *Good Health.* Logically, we consider the feasibility of checking out the STATUS OF AMERICAN HEALTH. Yes, why not? We will take a look at American Health to see if we can possibly find clues there.

STATUS OF AMERICAN HEALTH

Statistics show that America has a population more than 243 million. We are 5.1% of the world's population; yet, we control 25% of the world's wealth. We have more resources than any other country in the world.

In 1986, we spent 458.2 billion dollars on health care alone. This is 10.6% of our Gross National Product. The entire Gross National Product for many other countries around the world is less than 458.2 billion dollars. In other words, not only does the United States spend more on health care than any other country in the world, we spend more on health care than many other countries have to take care of all of their needs.

We live in one of the most technologically advanced countries in the world. Our technology (machines, instruments, etc.) far surpasses that in most countries the world over. As a matter of fact, our technicians have developed machines so complex that they can actually retrieve information for which doctors and experts in other fields have been unable to determine a use.

After reading the above information, one would naturally conclude that Americans would be the healthiest people on the face of planet earth. Sadly, this is far from true. We do not even rank in the top ten in relation to health care indicators.

Some of our sad statistics are listed below.

One-fourth (1/4) of our national work force has physical and emotional problems which are severe enough to interfere with job performance and cost our industries more than 200 million dollars a year.

One-third (1/3) of the nation's men die of heart disease before age 60 and 1/6 of our female population does the same.

We have 7.8 million people with Bronchitis.

Thirty-four million of us have High Blood Pressure.

There are 6,069,000 diagnosed diabetics and probably 5 million more people with the disease who don't even know it yet.

Eighty million of us are overweight. Thirty-one million of us are **more** than 30% above the ideal weight for our height and bone structure.

We have 10 million confirmed alcoholics in America.

Ninety-five per cent of our high school students have tried marijuana by the time they reach their senior year.

Six to eight percent of the nation's professionals are either drug addicts or alcoholics.

In our "ultra modern society" certain factors probably contribute heavily to these statistics. These factors are:

1.)   "Health Care" institutions focus primarily on:

- treatment rather than prevention.

- attempts to heal the physical being as if the mental and spiritual components do not exist.

2.)   As a general rule, we Americans tend to:

- take very little personal responsibility for maintaining our own health.

- look for treatment and cure rather than practicing preventive medicine.

■   try to block or ignore the fact that the human being is three-dimensional (mental, spiritual, and physical) rather than just physical.

■   have an attitude of "do as you please now, and worry about the consequences when they occur."

A few of our counter-productive health habits are:

■   One-hundred million Americans (70% of the adult population plus many teenagers and younger children) partake of alcoholic beverages on a regular basis.

■   It is a known fact that at least thirty seven million Americans are users of illegal drugs-- the true statistics are much higher. Drugs are so rampant in our society that it is difficult to accurately estimate the exact amount of use.

■   One-third of the adult population smokes and one-million teenagers pick up the habit each year.

■   Each day, Americans consume about three or four times as much salt, and almost twice as much protein as the body requires. We also partake of caffeine, processed foods, refined sugar, flour, and other substances which are not fit for human consumption.

What is even more alarming than the statistics themselves is the fact that all of the diseases and conditions presented on pages 28 and 29 are preventable. It has been recognized and documented that 75 - 80% of all physical and mental symptoms are a direct result of problems which are basically self-induced. In a few years, after more research has been done, we will be able to verify the fact that more than 95% of all health problems are directly related to counter-productive health habits which will either totally disappear or be greatly diminished with lifestyle adjustments.

As with all of the other information that we have gathered, studying the status of American Health has left us no closer to the location of the fountain that we seek than when we first began. So, we leave the Status of American Health and continue on our journey *IN SEARCH OF THE FOUNTAIN OF YOUTH.*

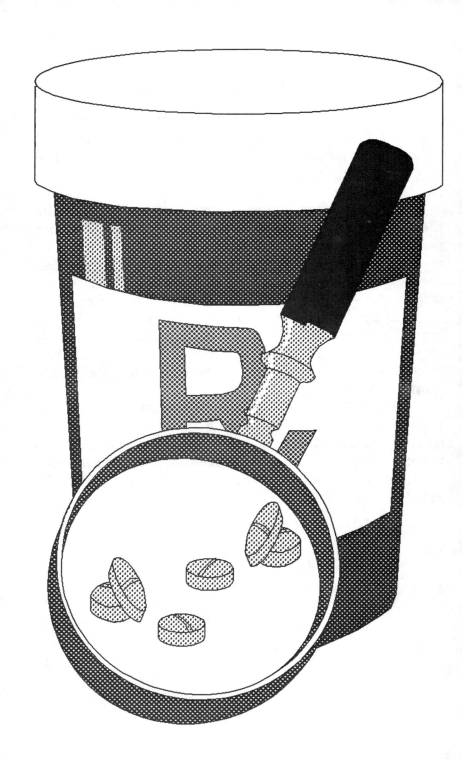

LEG 8

A SOAR THROUGH THE FIELD OF MEDICINE

S EARCHING through the Status of American Health gave us the idea about the next leg of our journey. We have decided to search the field of Medicine. We wonder why we didn't think of this in the beginning. If there is any group with helpful information, that group will be the people in the field of medicine. As we move through the search of the medical field, we note the dedication and sincere concern of some of the pioneers. They, unselfishly, gave their time, energy, and in some cases their very lives for the furtherance of medical science.

We rush through the mountains of documents, frequently stopping to pay attention to some particular diseases. Some very tragic diseases are listed below.

POLIOMYELITIS - (also known as infantile paralysis) is a contagious disease caused by a virus. It can progressively lead to paralysis and death. The earliest known documentation of this condition only dates back to the 18th century. There is a good chance that it existed prior to that time.

TUBERCULOSIS - is a contagious disease caused by a bacilli which usually attacks the lungs. Earlier, known as phthisis or consumption, it had a long deadly history until the mid 20th century.

SMALL POX - is an acute, often-fatal disease which moved through Europe during the 15th century. The various strains of the virus determined the deadliness of the condition.

CHOLERA - is another infectious disease caused by a bacterium which attacks the gastrointestinal tract. It most frequently occurs in epidemic outbreaks in areas where sanitary facilities are limited. In the 19th century, it was known to be in India for years. Later, it spread to many other parts of the world. It showed up in Europe in 1830 and had major outbreaks in 1848, 1854, 1865, and 1884. There was an epidemic in the United States between 1870 and 1873.

PLAGUE - has been definitely found to be the most dreadful of all of the contagious diseases. This condition, primarily spread by rodents, made its first known appearance over a thousand years ago among the Philistines. It has returned periodically to spread its venom and fear throughout numerous communities. By 100 A.D. it had appeared in Egypt, Libya, and Syria. It truly earned its nickname "**BLACK DEATH**" as it plowed through almost the entire world in 1347 and 1350. During this catastrophic period of time, the "**BLACK DEATH**" took the lives of one-fourth the men, women, and children of Europe.

As we continue our journey, wading through the medical journals and history books, we also become aware of other conditions such as **TYPHOID, TYPHUS, and MALARIA.**

During our exploration, we are mindful of the dedication of the leaders in the field of medicine. We note such names as Robert Koch, who discovered the cause of Cholera in 1884; and Sir Alexander Fleming, who discovered Penicillin in 1928. Also, the contributions of Jonas Salk, Edward Jenner, and Louis Pasteur do not go unnoticed.

As we sit back and marvel over the dedication of these people, we particularly note the contributions of Ignaz Philipp Semmelweis. Semmelweis was a Hungarian

Physician (1818 - 1865), who dealt with puerperal (child birth) fever. He observed that the death rate for women who delivered their babies in the hospital was much higher than the death rate for women who delivered at home.

Many times, medical students would perform autopsies and other pathological procedures; then, without washing their hands, they would examine one patient after another. They never stopped to wash their hands after procedures or between patients. In addition to his noticing that the death rate was higher for women who delivered in the hospital, Dr. Semmelweis noticed that patients with the highest death rates of all were those ladies who were attended by students who had just completed performing an autopsy. Semmelweis then insisted that all students under his charge wash their hands before examining any patient and between each patient. Even though this method resulted in an immediate drop in the maternal death rate for those women fortunate enough to be assigned to his care, all of Semmelweis' ideas were rejected and ridiculed.

We can feel the terrible torment and frustration that Semmelweis must have felt. Imagine, this dedicated, caring physician had actually, very dramatically, found the answer to this catastrophic problem--puerperal fever. He had found the key. He had a message to deliver to the medical world. We can almost hear him saying, "I have the answer, I know why these precious lives are being lost. I have proven my case but no one will listen to me." Yes, his reward for this brilliant discovery was rejection and ridicule from his colleagues.

In 1865, having been committed to a mental institution, Semmelweis closed his eyes in death. Several years after his death, hand-washing and other hygienic measures were incorporated into what is now accepted as sound, modern medical procedure. Oh, it is such a sad but true story. Semmelweis agonized over the problem until he found the answer. Then he agonized over the answer not being accepted to his own demise.

As we continue our search through the medical field, we read the information listed under "cause, treatment, healing, and prevention" for each of the diseases listed earlier in this leg of our journey. We notice that all of them have a lot in common. Each of the diseases was caused by a virus or bacteria, spread by insects, rodents, poor hygiene, lack of sanitary measures, poor or non-existent quarantine, or no isolation techniques. All of the health conditions which proved to be such catastrophic problems could have been prevented by the institution of simple sanitary and hygienic measures. Just imagine, something as simple as not your washing hands could cause such pain and suffering and have such a devastating effect on mankind.

As we ponder over the situation prior to the acceptance of hand-washing and other hygienic measures into medical practice, it is difficult to understand why these simple measures were so hard for medical practitioners to understand at that time. Of course, the point could easily be made that we understand the importance of hygiene in the context of 20th century medicine because we live in the 20th century. Practitioners of the 19th century had no way of knowing about these facts because this information simply was not available at that time. But as we continue our search, we become even more curious about these 19th century attitudes. There is documentation to show that proper sanitation and good hygienic measures were known and practiced thousands of years earlier. We really do need to explore this point further but we first need to understand two key pieces of information.

We need to understand:

■   what was happening medically when students examined women in the 19th century without washing their hands.

AND

■   why the death rate was so much greater for women attended by students who had just finished performing an autopsy.

The explanations for the above statements are as follow:

■   When a woman delivers a baby she discharges a substance called lochia. The lochia from one woman is extremely infectious to another patient.

■   A series of events take place when an animal (man or lower animal) dies. The blood stops circulating; thus, removing the method of controlling the growth of bacteria in the body. Blood and body fluids become stagnant. When this happens all of the constituents in blood and other body fluids render them a perfect host or medium for the growth of bacteria and other living creatures which cannot be seen with the naked eye. A short time after death, the body becomes extremely infectious.

In the 19th century, when medical students examined women who had just given birth, one after the other without washing their hands; they were simply transporting infectious lochia from one woman to the next. This led to a very high death rate among these women. But, when medical students finished an autopsy, then went directly to the maternity ward and began examining one woman after the other without ever stopping to wash their hands, it is easy to see why the death rate for these patients was the highest of all. The medical students were compounding the problem of transporting infectious lochia by adding to the lochia the bacteria and other microbes from a dead body.

While, it is truly mind-boggling to think that such a simple procedure as hand-washing could have saved so many lives, it is even more mind-boggling when we think that medical practitioners of the nineteenth century had no concept of this fact; yet, people who lived as early as 1490

B. C. were given definite instructions concerning hand-washing, hygiene, and sanitation. Interestingly, these instructions included precautions against touching dead bodies.

> "And the LORD spake unto Moses, saying,
> Speak unto the children of Israel, saying, If a woman have conceived seed, and born a man child: then she shall be unclean seven days; according to the days of the separation for her infirmity shall she be unclean."
> Leviticus 12:1-2

> "But if she bear a maid child, then she shall be unclean two weeks, as in her separation: and she shall continue in the blood of her purifying threescore and six days."
> Leviticus 12:5

Look what happens when we combine the three scriptures that follow with the two above.

"He that touched the dead body
of any man shall be unclean
seven days."
Numbers 19:11

"And whatsoever the unclean
person toucheth shall be
unclean; and the soul that
toucheth it shall be unclean
until even."
Numbers 19:22

"And the clean person shall
sprinkle upon the unclean on
the third day, and on the
seventh day: and on the
seventh day he shall purify
himself, and wash his clothes,
and bathe himself in water,
and shall be clean at even."
Numbers 19:19

When we put all of these scriptures together, we see
a very clear warning against the poor hygienic practices
which were common during the 19th century. During
Semmelweis' lifetime, the death rate for childbirth fever
was much higher in hospitals than in home deliveries
because infectious lochia was transferred from one woman
to another through unsterile techniques in hospitals. The
highest death rate of all was among those women attended
by medical students who had just completed performing an

autopsy. In such cases, filth was collected from the dead body and transferred to the helpless mothers. Yet, the scriptures warning against such practices were written in 1490 B.C. Semmelweis discovered the results of these improper hygienic methods and attempted to do something about them, but to no avail.

We began our journey through the field of medicine in hope of finding answers; yet, questions were raised. We saw true brilliance, concern, and dedication; but, it was rewarded with ridicule and rejection.

We are mindful of the fact that we are still no closer to the object of our search than when we first began. Yet, for the first time we have run into some material which is somewhat helpful to us. We feel a lot more encouraged than discouraged. So we reaffirm our dedication as we continue on our journey *IN SEARCH OF THE FOUNTAIN OF YOUTH.*

LEG 9

MODERN PROBLEMS - SAME OLD SOLUTIONS

A S we continue to look at the scriptures, we find information which addresses the same medical problems which affect our society today. Interestingly, there is a tremendous amount of evidence available which tells us that major advances identified as giant steps for medical science was information that was known centuries earlier and used by people of those times. Since our interest has been pricked, now is a good time to pause and look at some of this evidence. In Leg 8 of our journey we talked about sanitation and hygiene; so, let us continue on this course.

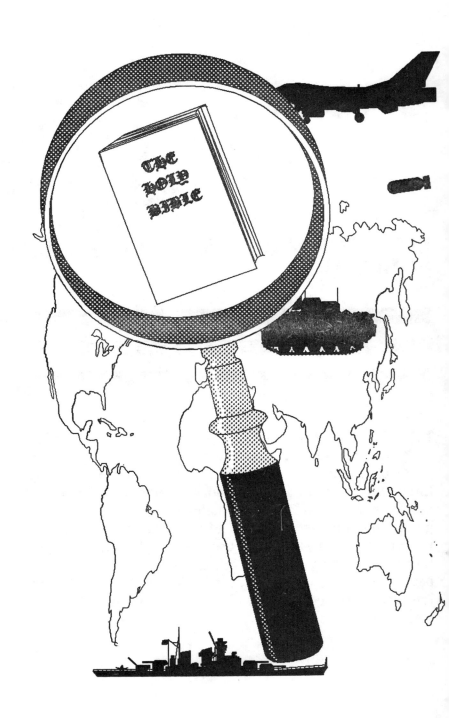

INFECTION CONTROL

Today all modern hospitals pay strict attention to infection control. With all of the research available, prompted by physicians of the 19th century, we **"NOW"** know how infectious diseases are transmitted. We are also **"NOW"** aware of the fact that the single most effective and important infection control method is proper hand-washing in running water.

Even though "modern" medical practitioners only learned about infection control in the 19th century, people who lived in 1490 B.C. already knew how infectious diseases were transmitted. They had definite instructions concerning proper sanitation, hygiene, and isolation techniques.

The most profound outbreak of Bubonic Plague occurred in 1347 A. D. We **"NOW"** know that it was due to the infestation of rodents which was, in turn, due to improper disposal of human waste. Yet, as early as 1451 B.C. (more than three thousand years ago) this scripture was given.

"Thou shalt have a place also without the camp, whither thou shalt go forth abroad: And thou shalt have a paddle upon thy weapon; and it shall be, when thou wilt ease thyself abroad, thou shalt dig

> therewith, and shalt turn back
> and cover that which cometh
> from thee:"

Deuteronomy 23:12-13

Proper sanitation includes proper disposal of human waste. This has proven to be another major factor in preventing communicable diseases. Other instructions on proper sanitation are cited in such scriptures as Leviticus 15:1-13.

Also, as early as 1140 B.C., the people already knew that the plague was caused by rodents. Once again, we find evidence of this fact in the scriptures.

> "Then said they, What shall be
> the trespass offering which we
> shall return to him? They
> answered, Five golden
> emerods, and five golden mice,
> according to the number of the
> lords of the Philistines: for one
> plague was on you all, and on
> your lords."
> "Wherefore ye shall make
> images of your emerods, and
> images of your mice that mar
> the land; and ye shall give
> glory unto the God of Israel;
> peradventure he will lighten his

hand from off you, and from
off your gods, and from off
your land."
I Samuel 6:4-6

Emerods are the same as buboes (the inflamed lymph glands which are a part of the disease process in the plagues) hence the other well known name for this condition, the "Bubonic Plague".

CHOLESTEROL

Another example of how the diseases and concerns of today are problems which were discussed and dealt with centuries ago, lies in the instructions given to avoid high cholesterol levels. Cholesterol is an organic, fatty compound which occurs naturally in the bodies of animals and is totally essential for life. Therefore, people--like other animals, manufacture their **_OWN_** cholesterol. It is synthesized internally by natural means and is dangerous only when levels become too high or too low.

Extremely low cholesterol levels may be an indication of malnutrition. In this country; however, the most frequently encountered problem of the two is cholesterol levels which are too high. The two main reasons that people develop high cholesterol levels are improper diet and excessive stress. When people eat flesh meat, extra cholesterol is taken into the system. During stressful reactions, the body goes through certain chemical reactions which result in an increase of blood cholesterol levels. High cholesterol levels are associated with heart disease, America's number-one health problem and number-one cause of death.

When high cholesterol levels are detected, the first thing that a physician recommends is a change in diet which includes a reduction in the amount of fat taken into the body. As early as 1490 B.C. people received instructions not to eat fat.

> "It shall be a perpetual statue for your generations throughout all your dwellings, that ye eat neither fat nor blood."
> Leviticus 3:17

SUBSTANCE ABUSE

We don't have to look far to find another major health problem in our ultra modern society--**CHEMICAL OR SUBSTANCE ABUSE.** Chemical or substance abuse can involve any substance which is capable of producing physical, mental, or emotional changes within the user. This problem has now become common among people of all ages, walks of life, and social and economic statuses in our society. We have explored numerous substances. A few of the more commonly used ones are listed below.

ALCOHOL - is a harmful chemical. It enters the blood stream from the stomach at a very rapid rate. Within minutes it has moved to all parts of the body.

In the early phases of intoxication, alcohol causes loss of judgment and efficiency. The intoxicated individual moves through several stages of emotional, erratic behavior. In severe cases an individual can become unable to speak coherently or walk. He or she runs the risk of losing consciousness or dying from respiratory arrest.

The National Council on Alcoholism estimates that there are some 100 million persons in this country over the age of 15 who are consumers of alcohol. Of these, there are an estimated 10 million people suffering from the disease alcoholism.

There is no "typical" alcoholic. Among men, drinking problems occur most frequently in the early twenties and in the thirties among women. Each year, about 100,000 drinkers develop alcoholism. The number of known women alcoholics has doubled since World War II.

Alcoholism ranks with cancer and heart disease as a major risk to the nation's health. Yet, it is the most neglected health problem in the United States. Deaths from cirrhosis of the liver, one of the complications of this dreadful disease, have increased 67% over the last 20 years.

Between six and ten percent of the nation's employees suffer from alcoholism. This statistic makes alcoholism a very expensive disease. Absenteeism, health and welfare services, property damage, and medical expenses are estimated to cost our nation's work forces around 25 billion dollars each year.

A large percentage of the problems of a catastrophic nature encountered on a regular basis are related to alcohol.

Fatal Accidents	50%
Fire Deaths	53%
Drownings	45%
Home Accidents	22%
Pedestrian Accidents	55%
Arrest by law enforcement officers	55%
Admissions to state/co. mental hospitals	37.4%
Murders	64%
Assaults	41%
Rapes	34%
Other Sex Crimes	29%
Suicides	30%
Domestic Violence	60%

Alcohol is a primary component in such drinks as wine, whiskey, beer, and certain medications.

In the 20th century, we realize that *ALCOHOL IS BAD NEWS.* Of course, as with all other information discussed, people received instructions concerning the negative effects of alcohol thousands of years ago. The following passage from Proverbs was written 1000 B.C.

> "Wine is a mocker, strong drink
> is raging: and whosoever is
> deceived thereby is not wise."
> Proverbs 20:1

Look at this same scripture in the Living Bible.

> "WINE GIVES FALSE, courage;
> hard liquor leads to brawls;
> what fools men are to let it
> master them, making them reel
> drunkenly down the street!"
> Proverbs 20:1

To some extent we are a little confused, we find scriptures which clearly state that many of the Biblical patriarchs drank wine.

> "And Noah began to be an
> husbandman, and he planted a
> vineyard;
> And he drank of the wine, and
> was drunken; and he was
> uncovered within his tent."
> Genesis 9:20,21

And what about this scripture? It seems to be the all-time favorite of those who want to make the point that the Bible says that alcoholic beverages are not only "okay", but really necessary for good health.

"Drink no longer water, but use a little wine for thy stomach's sake and thine often infirmities."
I Timothy 5:23

Also, frequently the point is made that not only did JESUS himself drink wine but he made it.

"And the third day there was a marriage in Cana of Galilee; and the mother of Jesus was there:
And both Jesus was called, and his disciples, to the marriage.
And when they wanted wine, the mother of Jesus saith unto him, They have no wine.
Jesus saith unto them, Fill the waterpots with water. And they filled them to the brim.
And he saith unto them, Draw out now, and bear unto the governor of the feast. And they bare it.
When the ruler of the feast had tasted the water that was made wine, and knew not whence it was: (but the servants which

> drew the water knew;) the
> governor of the feast called the
> bridegroom,
> And saith unto him, Every man
> at the beginning doth set forth
> good wine; and when men
> have well drunk, then that
> which is worse: but thou hast
> kept the good wine until now."

John 2:1-3,7-10

Our confusion on the issue of wine lasts but a little while as we continue our study of the Holy Scriptures and a few other books. We are presented with some interesting facts that clear this matter up for us. First, let us note that there is no place in the Scriptures where Jesus or any member of the Godhead condoned, made, or recommended intoxicating beverages. Yes, we are aware of the fact that there are Biblical texts that clearly state that the Patriarchs drank wine, Jesus drank and made wine, and Paul recommended the use of wine to Timothy. There is a very simple explanation.

Prior to the 20th century, the term *"WINE"* referred to the *"JUICE OF THE GRAPE" "FERMENTED OR UNFERMENTED"*. UNFERMENTED grape juice is a very healthy beverage. FERMENTED grape juice is the "mocker" referred to in Proverbs 20:1. All who partake of it are definitely "unwise".

Just how did this confusion about what "is" and "isn't" wine come about? Well, prior to 1905, all "juice of the grape" was referred to as "wine". In 1905 France passed a law that said "no drink may be kept or sold under the name **"VINO", (WINE)** that is not exclusively produced from the **FERMENTATION** of fresh grapes". In 1925 Italy passed a law which defined wine as "the product of **ALCOHOLIC FERMENTATION** of the juice of the grape whether slightly fresh or slightly dried". In 1930, Germany passed a law even more strict which definitely set "wine" apart as that which is **FERMENTED.**

Today, all the world refers to "wine" as a **FERMENTED ALCOHOLIC BEVERAGE.** The first law making this distinction was passed in France just 85 years ago. The Bible was written thousands of years ago when the term "wine" meant "juice of the grape", **FERMENTED** or **UNFERMENTED.**

The fact that at one time, "wine" meant "fermented" as well as "unfermented" is not at all unusual. One word having several meanings is a very familiar concept. We use them all of the time and think nothing of it. Such words are called **HOMONYMS.** A precious few of the more frequently used homonyms are: check, change, stage, cross, rash, bridge, stroke, and state. So, during Biblical times "wine" was used to refer to **fermented** and **unfermented** grape juice, just as "meat" meant fruits, nuts, and grains, in 4000 B.C. (See Genesis 1:29).

Now, we can stop saying that Jesus drank "wine" as we think of "wine" in 1991. And, of course, we know the next comment. If "wine" referred to "grape juice", why did Noah become drunken? The answer to this question is easy. Since in Biblical times "WINE" referred to both the fermented and unfermented grape juice; obviously, Noah drank the fermented version referred to in Proverbs 20:1.

OTHER COMMONLY USED DRUGS

MARIJUANA - commonly referred to as grass, pot, or weed is a plant which contains a major mind-altering ingredient (delta-9-tertahydrocannabionl, or THC). Over 400 other chemicals are contained in this one plant.

LSD - is a synthetic hallucinogen which was converted to LSD in 1938. Its mind-altering properties only became known in 1943.

PCP - commonly called "angel dust" is a drug which was developed for surgical use in the late 1850s. It can produce violent and bizarre behavior in people and may result in serious injury and even death.

COCAINE - is a very powerful drug extracted from the leaves of the coca plant. It can increase the heart rate and blood pressure and can trigger psychosis in users.

There are several scriptural references which let us know that thousands of years ago, people received warnings against the dangers of **"SUBSTANCE ABUSE"**.

> "Lest there should be among you man, or woman, or family, or tribe, whose heart turneth away this day from the LORD our God, to go and serve the gods of these nations; lest there should be among you a

root that beareth gall and wormwood."
Deuteronomy 29:18

"Wine is a mocker, strong drink is raging: and whosoever is deceived thereby is not wise."
Proverbs 20:1

"Woe unto him that giveth his neighbor drink, that puttest thy bottle to him, and makest him drunken also, that thou mayest look on their nakedness."
Habakkuk 2:15

"What? Know ye not that your body is the temple of the Holy Ghost which is in you, which ye have of God, and ye are not your own?"
"For ye are bought with a price: therefore glorify God in your body, and in your spirit, which are God's."
I Corinthians 6:19-20

"Whether therefore ye eat, or drink, or whatsoever ye do, do all to the glory of GOD."
I Corinthians 10:31

> "And be not drunk with wine,
> wherein is excess; but be filled
> with the Spirit;"

Ephesians 5:18

We are truly amazed. So much information related to medical practices simply shows that modern research has only served to "prove" what was already known. There is much more evidence to support this fact than that which has already been presented. Note the facts that follow.

INFANT DEVELOPMENT

During the first few days after birth, the newborn infant undergoes more rapid changes than at any other time during his or her entire life span. The most profound changes begin during labor and continue for approximately seven days after birth. All systems undergo dramatic changes, but of particular interest are the changes which occur in the circulatory system. The peripheral circulation is sluggish for the first one or two hours after birth. During this period the infant appears cyanotic or bluish. The pulse rate fluctuates between 100 and 180 depending on the activity level of the child at any given moment. The infant's blood pressure is characteristically low and gradually rises for about seven days. The concentration of erythrocytes and hemoglobin undergoes vast changes. Approximately one week after birth, these levels are equal to cord blood levels.

Immediately after birth the infant's intestinal tract does not contain the bacteria which are necessary for the synthesis of Vitamin K. Vitamin K is essential for the development of prothrombin and other coagulation factors which are important in the control of bleeding. In other words, the infant suffers from a transitory deficiency in blood coagulation factors between the 2nd and 5th day of his or her life outside the mother's womb. This condition spontaneously moves to normal in a few more days--by the seventh day to be exact. The concentration of the various white blood cells also goes through changes. By the end of the first week, the lymphocytes predominate. Lymphocytes are important in the formation of antibodies. Antibodies render us immune to certain foreign particles introduced into the blood stream.

Unless you are a member of the medical or nursing profession, you may have found the information presented above boring and difficult to understand. The whole point of the presentation was to denote the fact that *THERE IS A VERY BEST TIME TO PERFORM AN INVASIVE PROCEDURE ON A NEWBORN INFANT*--that time is on the *"EIGHTH DAY"*. A circumcision is an invasive procedure routinely performed on male infants. Typically, in modern hospitals physicians do not wait for the eighth day; therefore, they have to administer vitamin K artificially.

Scriptures clearly state that if a circumcision is going to be performed, it should be performed on the eighth day.

INSTRUCTIONS GIVEN TO ABRAHAM
APPROXIMATELY 1898 B. C.

"And he that is eight days old
shall be circumcised among
you,"
Genesis 17:12

Some of the other scriptures which deal with circumcision on the eighth day are listed below.

THE CIRCUMCISION OF ISAAC (ISRAEL) ON THE EIGHTH DAY

"And Abraham circumcised his
son Isaac being eight days old,
as God had commanded him."
Genesis 21:4

THE CIRCUMCISION OF THE CHILDREN OF ISRAEL ON THE EIGHTH DAY

"And the LORD spake unto
Moses saying,
"Speak unto the children of
Israel, saying, If a woman have
conceived seed, and born a
man child: then she shall be
unclean seven days; according
to the days of the separation

for her infirmity shall she be unclean.
"And in the eighth day the flesh of his foreskin shall be circumcised."
Leviticus 12:2

THE CIRCUMCISION OF JOHN THE BAPTIST ON THE EIGHTH DAY

"And it came to pass, that on the eighth day they came to circumcise the child; and they called him Zacharias, after the name of his father.
And his mother answered and said, Not so; but he shall be called John."
Luke 1:59-60

THE CIRCUMCISION OF JESUS ON THE EIGHTH DAY

"And when eight days were accomplished for the circumcising of the child, his name was called JESUS, which was so named of the angel

before he was conceived in the
womb."
Luke 2:21

PAUL ACKNOWLEDGES THAT HE WAS CIRCUMCISED ON THE EIGHTH DAY

"Circumcised the eighth day, of
the stock of Israel, of the tribe
of Benjamin, an Hebrew of the
Hebrews; as touching the law a
Pharisee;"
Philippians 3:5

COLON CANCER

A QUICK check of the health statistics will tell us that the incidence of colon cancer is on the rise. It has been determined that this unfortunate increase is directly related to poor eating habits (between meal snacks, overeating, and an increase in the intake of sugar and rich desserts). Scriptures were given thousands of years ago which warn against these counter productive health habits.

"When thou sittest to eat with
a ruler, consider diligently
what is before thee:
And put a knife to thy throat, if
thou be a man given to
appetite."

"Be not desirous of his dainties:
for they are deceitful meat."
Proverbs 23:1-3

"For the drunkard and the
glutton shall come to poverty:
and drowsiness shall clothe a
man with rags."
Proverbs 23:21

"It is not good to eat too much
honey:..."
Proverbs 25:27

BLOOD CIRCULATION

William Harvey (1578-1657) is credited with discovering the circulation of the blood in the human body. His discovery is said to have revolutionized medical science. Prior to Harvey's work concerning the circulation of the blood, medical practitioners had no idea of the importance of blood to life itself. Yet, the scripture below was given 1490 B. C.

"For the life of the flesh is in
the blood:..."
Leviticus 17:11

EMPIRICAL VERSUS SCIENTIFIC RESEARCH

As we move through this vast amount of material, we run across the term "**EMPIRICAL**" which refers to a certain method of learning. The history books tell us that this is the only method that scientists had to learn about the world in which they lived prior to the 19th century. Empiricism is a method of observation in which results are accepted without controlling the variables. Scientific research is the method used by researchers today. Since we have become sophisticated enough to control the variables in an experiment, we can be sure that our results are not influenced by something which escapes our observation. This helps us to be sure that our results are accurate. This procedure involves the following:

- establishing or writing a hypothesis.

- establishing a control group and a scientific group (this is necessary to control the variables being observed).

- performing the experiment for a specified period of time.

- checking the results.

AND THEN

■   accepting or rejecting the hypothesis set forth in the first step of this procedure.

The implementation of scientific research is obviously the turning point toward progress and modernization. It is a concept which mostly developed during the early years of the 20th century. Textbooks state that 90% to 95% of the information which constitutes the bodies of knowledge of all modern fields was discovered during the last 50 to 70 years. Ninety percent of the individuals who made these discoveries are still alive today.

Even though scientific research, according to the writers of scientific history, is a totally modern concept; Daniel, the Old Testament Prophet, used these principles as early as 607 B.C.

Biblical history records the fact that Daniel was in captivity in Babylon. As in all cases in which people are taken into captivity; conquerors tend to select the strongest, healthiest, and smartest looking people to do special kinds of work. They also tend to do the things that they feel will enhance the strength and health of the captives. This was done to obtain the best possible service.

So Nebuchadnezzar, the King of Babylon, believing as do many people today, that meat and wine make one stronger and healthier, decided that the children of Israel would be of greater service to him if he fed them better.

"And the king appointed them a daily provision of the king's meat, and of the wine which he drank: so nourishing them

> three years, that at the end
> thereof they might stand before
> the king."

Daniel 1:5

Daniel, being vegetarian and a child of God, knew that the simple vegetarian diet was healthier. So, he decided that he did not want the diet that the king offered.

> "But Daniel purposed in his
> heart that he would not defile
> himself with the portion of the
> king's meat, nor with the wine
> which he drank:..."

Daniel 1:8

Daniel found himself in a special predicament, he couldn't just tell the king, "No, thanks, I don't want to eat flesh meat and drink (fermented) wine". So Daniel had to get permission to prove his point. He performed a "modern day" experiment using **"SCIENTIFIC RESEARCH"**.

> Prove thy servants, I beseech
> thee, ten days; and let them
> give us pulse to eat, and water
> to drink."

Daniel 1:12

Daniel's
Hypothesis: A diet of pulse (the edible parts of leguminous plants such as beans, peas, etc.) and water is much healthier than a diet of flesh meat and wine.

Research
Group: The members of the research group were Daniel and the three Hebrew boys: Hananiah, Mishael, and Azariah (these three young men are better known as Shadrach, Meshach, and Abednego).

Control
Group: The king's men and certain Israelites who consumed wine and flesh meats.

Experiment
time: Ten days.

Experiment
Results: Accept the hypothesis. The vegetarian diet (pulse and water) was proven to be much healthier.

> "And at the end of ten days their countenances appeared fairer and fatter in flesh than all the children which did eat the portion of the king's meat."
Daniel 1:15

WE ARE STILL ON OUR MISSION

We have spent a great deal of time comparing modern medicine and science to ancient information. Have we forgotten our mission? No, we are still **IN SEARCH OF THE FOUNTAIN OF YOUTH.** But, we are running into information that is so fascinating, we just want to linger for a while longer. Shortly, we will resume our journey **IN SEARCH OF THE FOUNTAIN OF YOUTH.** But before we go, let's look at a few more informational gems.

FIRST SURGERY

On December 13, 1809, Dr. Ephraim McDowell performed what is believed to be the first ovariotomy. His patient, Mrs. Jane Todd Crawford, recited from Psalms throughout the procedure. The medical history books provide us with a descriptive picture of Mrs. Crawford's post-operative (recovery) period. The entire series of events was a remarkable feat for patient and physician.

Dr. McDowell operated during the pre-anaesthetic, pre-antiseptic, and almost even the pre-surgical era. After he performed the procedure on Mrs. Crawford, Dr. McDowell went on to perform several more operations; subsequently, becoming recognized worldwide for his great accomplishments. Even though it is known that he was not the first person to perform a surgical procedure, Dr. McDowell is considered a really great pioneer who made a substantial contribution to the field of medicine.

As we continue our search, we are amazed that we can actually locate the very first surgery that was performed on planet earth. Again we find it recorded in the Bible. It occurred around 4004 B.C. with Adam as the patient and God, the Master Physician, performing the operation.

> "And the LORD caused a deep sleep to fall upon Adam, and Adam slept: and he took one of his ribs, and closed up the flesh instead thereof;"
> Genesis 2:21

Notice that God did not need antibiotics or anesthesia and Adam needed no period of time to recover. *"WHAT A MIGHTY GOD WE SERVE."*

VEGETARIANISM: FACT OR FAD

Today people are really becoming more "health conscious". All over America we hear, "cut down on red meat, eat more bran, certain kinds of fish reduce cholesterol, fiber in the diet is good for you", ad infinitum. Actually, this all sounds like good advice. One thing that concerns us is the fact that **ADVICE** is so changeable. Today we are told that something is good for us, tomorrow there is a recall of that same item because it has been found to cause cancer or some other dreaded disease.

There is a current trend in which more and more people are moving towards vegetarianism for improved health. Then, there are others who swear that "flesh" meat is necessary in order for us to obtain adequate protein. So, what about vegetarianism, is it really healthier or is it just another "fad" that people are going through? Well, let's take a look at the evidence.

FACT # 1. Anatomical studies have been done on animals which divide them into categories based on the structure of the mouth, teeth, and digestive tract. They are then labeled according to the type food that their systems can tolerate. The three categories are:

a.   Carnivores - flesh meat eaters

b.   Herbivores - vegetarians

c.   Omnivores - mostly vegetarian but flesh meat may be included in the diet.

People are not designed exactly like any of the animals, but it has been established that people are more similar to the herbivores than the other two categories. We definitely know that we are not carnivores; omnivores--maybe, but that becomes very doubtful as we look at the other evidence available.

FACT # 2. "The adequacy of a diet containing little or no flesh meat was put to the test in Denmark during World War I. Because of the allied blockade of imports, the government was afraid that there would be a critical shortage of food. It asked Denmark's vegetarian society and Dr. Mikkel Hindheds, a strong advocate of simple living, to organize the rationing program. The Danish people came through the war with **IMPROVED HEALTH** and lowered death rates although eating primarily whole grain and bran bread, barley, porridge, potatoes, greens, and dairy products."

FACT # 3. "Norway went through a similar experience during World War II. From 1940 to 1945 their consumption of animal products was drastically cut, and the use of cereals, potatoes, and other vegetables was increased. Deaths from circulatory diseases were considerably fewer during this period of time. With the end of the war; however, the people returned to their prewar diet and the death rate promptly rose to prewar levels."

Facts #2 and #3 were taken from the magazine, "Life and Health", Volume 1, Second Edition; Vegetarianism: A New Concept page 9.

As a result of extensive research after World War II (after 1945), we know that vegetarians, as a group, have fewer diseases and live an average of 10-12 years longer than people who eat flesh meat.

FACT # 4. We knew that we would eventually have to come back to our favorite reference book (The Holy Bible) to further verify our findings.

Return with us now, to those thrilling days of yesteryear and let us explore the Old Testament. Take a look at **THIS** astounding observation. From the time of Adam to the time of Noah accounts for nine generations. *FROM ADAM TO NOAH THE AVERAGE AGE AT DEATH WAS 912 YEARS.* From Shem, (one of Noah's sons) to Abraham accounts for ten generations. *DURING THIS PERIOD OF TIME THE AVERAGE AGE AT DEATH DROPPED FROM 912 YEARS TO 317 YEARS.* Adam lived 930 years and Noah was 950 when he died. Shem lived to be 600 years old and Abraham was 175 when he died. Moses lived to be 120 years old (Deuteronomy 34:7), and Joshua died at age 110 (Joshua 24:29).

At the death of Moses in 1451 B. C. and Joshua in 1427 B. C., the average age at death was about 70 years--very close to what it is today. We have been trained to believe that people who inhabited the earth thousands of years ago had a much shorter life span than people living today. Actually, this is not true. Man's life span has continuously been reduced since the flood. It seemed to taper off at about seventy during Moses' life time. This is truly amazing, in Genesis 6:3, God said that man would not live past 120 years. With all of our modern, medical discoveries and advances, it is still almost unheard of for anyone to live past

120 years. In reality the human race has made no progress toward increasing the quality and quantity of life since God used Moses to part the Red Sea. It was God's intention that man's life span be allowed to shorten. It seems that God used the flood as the dividing point to accomplish this goal.

A close study of the scriptures reveals that the only significant difference between pre-flood and post-flood lifestyles among the patriarchs was the introduction of flesh meat into the diet. If we took time to study all of the available research which proves that vegetarians live longer than flesh eaters, we would truly be astounded. But, modern research is but a minute replication of the remarkable testimony of the Old Testament.

FACT # 5. The most dramatic and important fact that should really clear up the confusion about vegetarianism once and for all (believe it or not) is a direct statement from The Bible made by none other than the Creator of the universe Himself, GOD.

> "And GOD said, Behold, I have given you every herb bearing seed, which is upon the face of all the earth, and every tree, in the which is the fruit of a tree yielding seed; to you it shall be for meat."
> Genesis 1:29

"...and thou shalt eat the herb of the field:"
Genesis 3:18

WELLNESS (HEALTH MAINTENANCE/ENHANCEMENT)

As we continue our search, we find that such fields of study as **Wholistic Health, Holistic Health, Stress Management, Preventive Medicine, Wellness, Natural Healing,** and **Physical Fitness** are subjects of constant discussion. We note that there is similar and overlapping information in all of these topics. We are also hasty to recognize the fact that a great deal of this information is very interesting and if followed, it really does have amazingly positive effects upon our state of health. Since there are more similarities than differences, we will group all of this information under the general heading **"HEALTH MAINTENANCE/ENHANCEMENT"** or the more popular term WELLNESS.

We have pooled all of the information that we have gathered from the various books and articles on health maintenance/enhancement and stated it in our own words. Health is defined as a positive state of being in which an individual is the best that he or she can be **PHYSICALLY, MENTALLY, AND SPIRITUALLY.** Health maintenance is an active process which **CANNOT** be dealt with in a passive manner. This means that one has to consciously and actively do things to increase his or her chances of developing and maintaining a positive state of health. We pick up the fact that it is more cost effective in terms of financial, physical, spiritual, emotional, and mental suffering, and wasted time to do certain things up front, rather than wait until sickness occurs then work on a cure.

Very notable contributions in the field of health maintenance come from the pens of pioneers George Westberg and Dr. Lester Breslow. When Westberg started America's first wholistic health clinic at Good Shepherd Lutheran Church in Springfield, Ohio in 1970, he hoped that the idea would rapidly spread. And it has spread; though, not as rapidly as it should have considering the benefits to be gained. We Americans lag far behind in relation to the concepts of "**taking responsibility for our own health**" and "**prevention is better than cure**". Even as late as the 1990s, many people still feel that they should eat, drink, and do whatever they wish; when, and however they desire, and worry about illness when it comes.

The concept of **WELLNESS** may be new to us "ultra" modern Americans, but (yes, you guessed correctly) the Holy scriptures show that Wellness was also known many centuries ago--as early as 1491 B.C. to be exact. Let us compare the following scripture from Exodus with our definition of wellness.

"And said, If thou wilt diligently hearken to the voice of the LORD thy GOD, and wilt do that which is right in his sight, and wilt give ear to his commandments, and keep all his statues, I will put none of

these diseases upon thee,
which I have brought upon the
Egyptians: for I am the LORD
that healeth thee."
Exodus 15:26

A tremendous amount of time and energy has been spent comparing the Bible to medical science. During our search in this area we ran across this excellent quote by Ellen G. White.

"SINCE the book of nature and the book of Revelation bear the impress of the same master mind, they cannot but speak in harmony. By different methods, and in different languages, they witness to the same great truths. Science is ever discovering new wonders; but she brings from her research nothing that, rightly understood, conflicts with divine revelation. The book of nature and the written word shed light upon each other. They make us acquainted with God by teaching us something of the laws through which He works."
Education page 128.

Reluctantly, we leave our "comparative analysis" of Medical Science and the Holy Bible. As always in the past, we have picked up a lot of information which is interesting and helpful. Yet, we must move on because we are still *IN SEARCH OF THE FOUNTAIN OF YOUTH.*

IN SEARCH *OF*
THE FOUNTAIN OF YOUTH

Section II.

THE FOUNTAIN
LOCATED

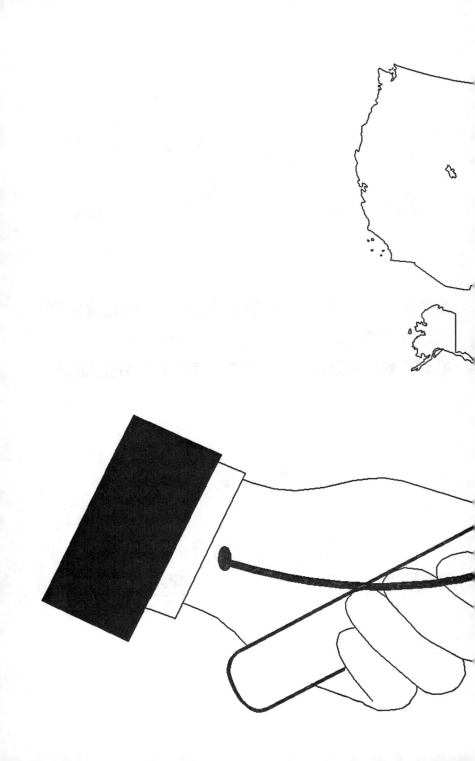

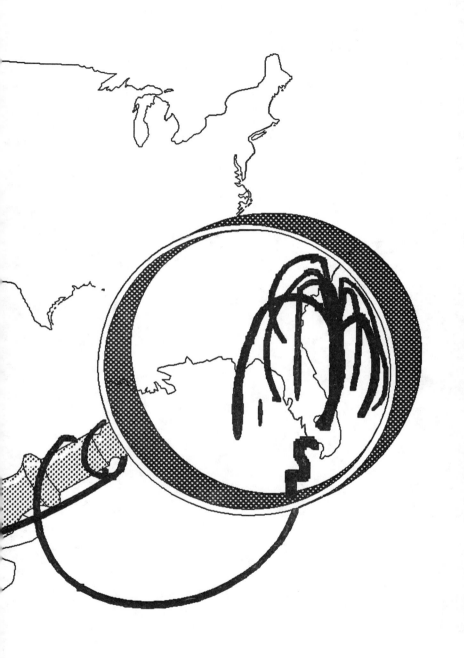

LEG 10

CAN YOU BELIEVE IT: WE ACTUALLY FIND THE
"FOUNTAIN OF YOUTH"

W E have searched through dictionaries, history books, encyclopedias, text books, medical journals, magazines, other professional journals, and even newspapers. We have looked at fountains, architecture, engineering, technology, scientific research, and medicine. We have explored the Status of American Health and searched parts of the Bible. At this point we still have not located the Fountain Of Youth, but we are no longer able to say that we are no closer to our destination than when we first began. We have picked up a tremendous amount of helpful information about health and well-being. Even though we have learned information from several sources, we acknowledge the fact that the one source of information which has stood the test of time is the Bible. At this point it is evident that medical science and Biblical Scriptures are, in essence, saying the same things. Of course, one can't help but notice that **THE BIBLE IS RUNNING ABOUT** *SIX THOUSAND YEARS AHEAD OF MEDICAL SCIENCE.* It seems as if God, through His infinite wisdom, has **ALLOWED** man to experiment with information that was already known and "**PROVE**" that it was correct.

These are truly amazing revelations but we have not forgotten our mission. We are still *IN SEARCH OF THE FOUNTAIN OF YOUTH.* So where do we go from here; it seems that there is no place left to be searched. Realizing that even the most astute detectives miss important evidence from time to time, maybe we should digress a little and look over the information that we have already packed away. Two important facts immediately come to us. First, we consider the fact that the Bible is the one source that has stood the test of time. Second, we look again at the fact that we have only searched **parts** of the Bible.

Question: "Should we continue our search of the Bible?"

Answer: A resounding, "**WHY NOT?**"

SEARCHING THE BIBLE FOR THE FOUNTAIN OF YOUTH

Before we go too far with this idea of continuing to search the Bible, we first need to know if we have permission to "search" the Bible. After all, this is God's Holy Word. So, out with the concordance; we'll start with the word "search". If we are given permission, we will then move to a few other words. Immediately, we find an open invitation to search the scriptures.

"Search the scriptures; for in them ye think ye have eternal life: and they are they which testify of me."
John 5:39

Did you notice that the above scripture mentions eternal life? If we find the FOUNTAIN OF YOUTH, is it possible that we will also receive information about eternal life? At this point, that is just "food for thought". Let us continue on our journey.

"If any of you lack wisdom, let him ask God, that giveth to all men liberally, and upbraideth not; and it shall be given him."
James 1:5

> "Call unto me, and I will answer thee, and shew thee great and mighty things, which thou knowest not."
> Jeremiah 33:3

We are tantalized as we begin our exploration through the Holy Scriptures **IN SEARCH OF THE FOUNTAIN OF YOUTH.** Along with our invitation to search, we are even given helpful instructions on how to search.

> "Whom shall he teach knowledge? and whom shall he make to understand doctrine? them that are weaned from the milk and drawn from the breasts."
> For precept must be upon precept, precept upon precept; line upon line, line upon line; here a little, and there a little:"
> Isaiah 28:9-10

The above scripture simply tells us how we have to study in order to discover the full meaning of this valuable information from the Bible. We usually have to look at the particular topic in several different texts and make comparisons and compile the various meanings for complete understanding. This is done under the guidance of the Holy Spirit.

Now, back to the Bible concordance. We will start in a fashion that is similar to how we started Leg 1 of our original journey--looking at **FOUNTAINS**.   There are 48 references to **FOUNTAINS** in the Old and New Testaments combined. We are particularly interested in the texts that follow.

"And if a man shall lie with a woman having her sickness, and shall uncover her nakedness; he hath discovered her fountain, and she hath uncovered the fountain of her blood: and both of them shall be cut off from among their people."
Leviticus 20:18

"And a certain woman, which had an issue of blood twelve years,
And had suffered many things of many physicians, and had spent all that she had, and was nothing bettered, but rather grew worse,
When she had heard of Jesus, came in the press behind, and touched his garment.
For she said, If I may touch but his clothes, I shall be whole.

> And straightway the fountain
> of her blood was dried up; and
> she felt in her body that she
> was healed of that plague."
Mark 5:25-29

Can you believe it, the Bible refers to the blood as a **FOUNTAIN**. Could the blood have anything to do with..? Now we are really intrigued. We need to study other scriptures relating to blood and see what we come up with. There are more than 350 references in the Bible which relate to blood. Several of them really make a strong impact.

> "For the life of the flesh is in
> the blood: and I have given it
> to you upon the altar to make
> an atonement for your souls:
> for it is the blood that maketh
> an atonement for the soul."
Leviticus 17:11

> "For it is the life of all flesh;
> the blood of it is for the life
> thereof: therefore I said unto
> the children of Israel, Ye shall
> eat the blood of no manner of
> flesh: for the life of all flesh is
> the blood thereof: whosoever
> eateth it shall be cut off."
Leviticus 17:14

"Only be sure that thou eat not the blood: for the blood is the life; and thou mayest not eat the life with the flesh."
Deuteronomy 12:23

When we put all of these scriptures together, using Biblical instructions (line upon line and precept upon precept; here a little and there a little), we can see two facts of major importance.

■ **THE BLOOD IS A FOUNTAIN.**

■ **THE BLOOD IS THE <u>LIFE</u> OF THE FLESH.**

With intense excitement, we return to the information that we gathered on Leg 1 at the beginning of our journey to make comparative notes. We look at the notes that explain exactly what we are looking for.

■   A substance which is a liquid.

■ **BLOOD IS A LIQUID.**

■   A liquid which is in constant motion.

■ **BLOOD IS IN CONSTANT MOTION.**

■ This liquid moves under pressure through something similar to pipes, conduits, or aqueducts.

■ **BLOOD MOVES UNDER PRESSURE THROUGH "PIPES, CONDUITS, AND AQUEDUCTS" CALLED BLOOD VESSELS (ARTERIES, VEINS, ARTERIOLES, VENULES, AND CAPILLARIES).**

■ This liquid, under normal circumstances, is covered.

■ **BLOOD IS COVERED BY "PIPES, CONDUITS, AND, AQUEDUCTS" CALLED BLOOD VESSELS (ARTERIES, VEINS, ARTERIOLES, VENULES, AND CAPILLARIES).**

■ This special liquid could even be some type of body fluid.

■ **BLOOD IS A BODY FLUID.**

■ Under ideal circumstances, this solution has the capability of giving us the feeling and appearance of being vigorous, lively, fresh, and active. And of course, it renders us free from diseases.

■ **IF AN INDIVIDUAL HAS HEALTHY BLOOD, SHE OR HE WILL BE VIGOROUS, FRESH, LIVELY, ACTIVE AND FREE FROM DISEASE.**

We remember the cliche, "I went searching for my happiness, only to find it in my own backyard". Well, we started a journey *IN SEARCH OF THE FOUNTAIN OF YOUTH* and found it even closer than our own backyards. Our search has lead us to the conclusion that we were carrying *A FOUNTAIN OF YOUTH* with us the entire time. Each of us is carrying a <u>FOUNTAIN OF YOUTH</u> within our very own bodies in our blood vessels. THE FOUNTAIN OF YOUTH IS THE BLOOD.

We have located the *FOUNTAIN OF YOUTH* only to realize that our mission is only half-completed. We understand that the *FOUNTAIN OF YOUTH* functions as a FOUNTAIN OF YOUTH only under certain circumstances-- when we have HEALTHY BLOOD. Now we will begin a journey IN SEARCH OF HEALTHY BLOOD.

We won't despair because we did learn from our previous search that we can eliminate a lot of the places that we have already searched and just go straight to the most helpful resource that we have found thus far--THE HOLY BIBLE.

IN SEARCH *OF*

THE FOUNTAIN OF YOUTH

Section III.

RESUMING OUR JOURNEY:
IN SEARCH OF THE
HEALTH LAWS

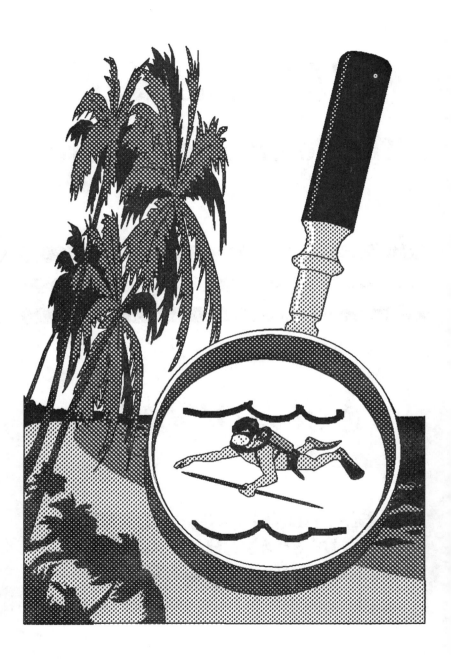

LEG 11

RESUMING OUR JOURNEY:
WE NEED MORE FACTS

W E are resuming our journey, only this time we are in search of what it takes to have healthy blood. Before we determine what makes healthy blood, it is necessary to gain an understanding of why blood is *"THE LIFE OF THE FLESH"*. To do this we must have a basic knowledge of *"THE FLESH"* (the human body). We will start with an overall review of the human system.

93

THE HUMAN DESIGN

The human system is specifically designed to exist in three components. The three components of human existence are:

- **SPIRITUAL**
- **MENTAL**
- **PHYSICAL**

Each component has five requirements which must be fulfilled in order to maintain the health and well-being of the whole person. These requirements are:

- **Nourishment.**
- **Exercise.**
- **Rest and relaxation.**
- **Elimination of waste from the system.**
- **Abstinence from all injurious substances or elements.**

All three components of the system require certain things in certain amounts. When we live counter to the specific design; the tissues and organs become strained causing them to malfunction, change structure in order to accommodate the extra burden, die prematurely, or develop damaged chromosomes, which can be passed on to our offspring. It can truthfully be said that all diseases result from:

- having something in the system that does not belong.

- not having something in the system which does belong.

- having certain things in the system in improper ratios and volumes.

No disease or condition just shows up from **"OUT OF NOWHERE."**

"As the bird by wandering, as the swallow by flying, so the curse causeless shall not come."
Proverbs 26:2

THE HUMAN PHYSICAL DESIGN

According to medical science, the human body is composed of 11 major systems.

I.   CIRCULATORY

a. Organs: Blood, Heart, Blood vessels, Spleen

b. Functions: distributes oxygen and nutrients to the
                          cells
                       removes CO_2 from the cells
                       removes waste from the cells
                       maintains Acid/Base balance
                       protects against diseases
                       helps regulate temperature

II.   INTEGUMENTARY

a. Organs: Hair, Skin, Fingernails, Sweat/Oil glands

b. Functions: regulates body temperature to protect the
                  body from foreign invasions
               eliminates waste
               synthesizes Vitamin D
               perceives stimuli (temperature, pressure,
                  and pain)

III.   SKELETAL

a. Organs: Bones, Cartilages, Joints

b. Functions: supports the body
                  protects the body
                  provides leverage
                  produces blood cells
                  stores nutrients

IV. MUSCULAR

a. Organs: All of the muscles of the body (skeletal, cardiac, visceral)

b. Functions: provides movement
maintains posture
provides facial expressions
produces heat

V. NERVOUS

a. Organs: Brain, Spinal Cord, certain of the sensory organs (ears, eyes)

b. Functions: regulates body impulses

VI. ENDOCRINE

a. Organs: All glands which produce hormones (pineal, pituitary, thyroid, parathyroids, thymus, adrenals, stomach, pancreas, small intestines, ovaries, testes)

b. Functions: regulates body activities through hormones transmitted via blood vessels

VII. **LYMPHATIC**

a. Organs: Lymph Nodes, Thoracic Ducts, Thymus, Spleen, Lymph vessels

b. Functions: returns proteins and plasma to the cardiovascular system
transports fats from the digestive system
filters the blood
produces white blood cells
protects against diseases

VIII. **RESPIRATORY**

a. Organs: Lungs, Pharynx, Trachea, Nasal cavity, Oral cavity, Larynx, Bronchus

b. Functions: supplies oxygen to the cells
eliminates Carbon dioxide
helps regulate acid/base balance

IX. **DIGESTIVE**

a. Organs: Mouth, Pharynx, Salivary glands, Esophagus, Liver, Gallbladder, Stomach, Pancreas, Small intestines, Large intestine, Rectum, Anus

b. Functions: performs physical/chemical
      breakdown of food
     eliminates waste

X. **URINARY**

 a. Organs: Kidneys, Urinary bladder, Urethra,
     Ureters

 b. Functions: regulates the chemical composition of
      the blood
     eliminates waste
     regulates fluid volume
     regulates electrolyte balance
     regulates acid/base balance

XI. **REPRODUCTIVE**

 a. Organs: (Male) Prostate gland, Vas deferens,
       Penis,
    (Female) Uterus, Ovaries, Vagina,
       Ovarian tubes

 b. Functions: perpetuates the species
    **CONTRARY TO POPULAR BELIEF, THIS
    SYSTEM HAS ABSOLUTELY <u>NO</u> FUNCTION
    IN MAINTAINING OR SUSTAINING THE
    INDIVIDUAL'S QUALITY OR
    QUANTITY OF LIFE.**

Each system is composed of organs. Each organ is composed of tissue. All tissue are composed of cells. The human body is composed of billions and billions of cells, most of which are much too small to be seen with THE NAKED EYE. All of the work of the body is performed at the cellular level. In other words, all of the work is performed by the cells.

EXAMPLE. The heart is an organ which is a part of the circulatory and muscular systems. It is composed of cardiac muscle tissue which is composed of millions of cells. The cardiac muscle cells change shape periodically (stretch and contract) to perform the duties of the heart muscle; to pump oxygenated blood to all of the billions of cells of the body. In order for the heart to perform as designed, each cardiac muscle cell must perform a certain amount of work coordinated with all of the other cells in the heart. When a small group of cells do not work properly, the heart will not work properly.

The work of all of the cells of the body is accomplished through a very complicated process of chemical reactions. All chemical reactions result in end-products or waste materials which must be removed from the cells. Cells are able to work properly only when two very important things occur:

■ they receive the correct nourishment which gives them the energy that they need to do their work.

■   end-products or waste materials are removed from the cells at a rapid and continuous rate.

When either one or both of these things are missing, the cells become sluggish and can malfunction or die prematurely. The blood is the life of the flesh because **NOURISHMENT** is carried to the cells by the blood and most of the **WASTE** is removed from the cells by the blood. The healthier the blood the more efficiently it does its job.

HEALTHY BLOOD

The Psalmist said, "I am fearfully and wonderfully made", (Psalms 139:14). Nowhere in the human system is this fact more dramatically illustrated than in the blood.

Since healthy blood is essential for a healthy body; it is therefore, essential to determine very specifically what healthy blood consists of and what it takes to obtain it.

MISCELLANEOUS INFORMATION ABOUT BLOOD

■   The blood is basically composed of Red Blood Cells (RBCs), the various White Blood Cells (WBCs), and plasma (the liquid which bathes the cells).

■   Red Blood Cells live for approximately 120 days.

■   The life of the average White Blood Cell ranges from a few hours to a few days.

- On the average, each millimeter (mm) of blood contains 4.8 million RBCs in women and 5.4 million RBCs in men.

- There are 5,000 to 9,000 WBCs per mm of blood.

THE BASIC FUNCTIONS OF BLOOD ARE TO:

- transport oxygen and other nutrients to the cells.

- transport waste material (end products of metabolism) away from the cells.

- transport specific hormones to specified glands. This function is essential for many bodily functions to occur.

- provide protection for the body by combating infection.

CHARACTERISTICS OF HEALTHY BLOOD

Healthy Blood:

- moves at a certain speed and pressure which is normal for the individual's age, sex, and weight.

- contains certain chemicals in very exact proportions.

- is able to transport an adequate supply of oxygen to the tissues.

- exists in a perfect balance between the WBCs, RBCs, specified chemicals, and the serum.

- flows through healthy vessels which have no abnormal blocks or strictures and have an adequate amount of elasticity".

- has a PH which is slightly alkaline.

- is adequate in volume.

- <u>MUST</u> be *FREE FROM ALL SUBSTANCES WHICH DO NOT NORMALLY BELONG IN THE BLOOD: (EXCESS HORMONES, CHEMICALS, CO_2 AND WASTE WHICH OCCURS WHEN FLESH MEAT IS A PART OF THE DIET.)*

We now know the requirements and components of HEALTHY BLOOD. Next, we will search the scriptures to find out what we can do to obtain healthy blood.

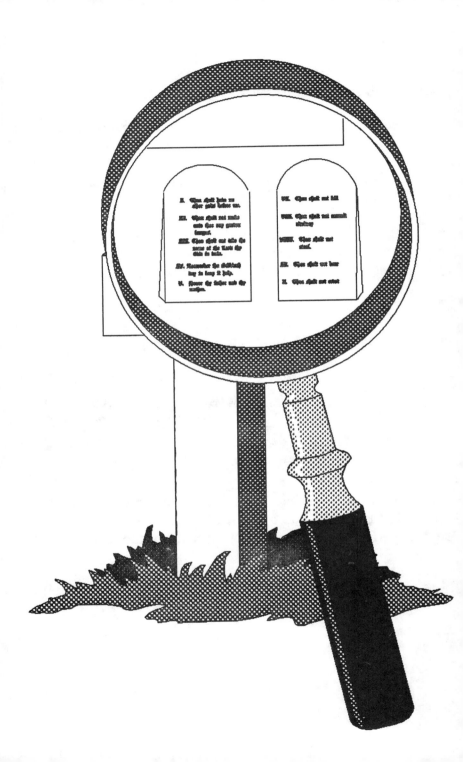

LEG 12

THE HEALTH LAWS: EMBEDDED IN GOD'S CHARACTER

T HE journey that we started **IN SEARCH OF THE FOUNTAIN OF YOUTH** landed us right in the middle of the Holy Scriptures. We readily acknowledge the fact that there has been more useful information received from the Bible than any other source that was searched. So we will look to the scriptures to complete our journey and find out how to have healthy blood.

Anything that comes from God exemplifies <u>HIS</u> character. Therefore, before we begin reciting health laws from the scriptures, we need to look at God's character. If it does not reflect His character, it's not from God.

IN SEARCH OF GOD'S CHARACTER

How do we check out the character of God? Well, God will allow us to learn of Him through the Bible. This is done by exploring that which was written **BY** God and that which was written **ABOUT** God.

Our exploration reveals that the Bible was written by approximately 40 men who were moved by the Spirit of God (II Peter 1:21) over a period of approximately 1600 years. It is composed of two major sections, The Old and New Testaments. Together these two sections contain 3,566,480 letters, 773,692 words, 31,173 verses, 1,189 chapters and 66 books. The Old Testament begins with the book of Genesis and the New Testament ends with the book of Revelation.

We find information related to: abortion (Exodus 21:22), the use of abusive language (Exodus 21:17 & Leviticus 19:14), and gossiping (Leviticus 19:16). There are over 150 statements which admonish people to care for the poor.

In the New Testament we find that Jesus quoted the Old Testament more than twenty times. There are about seventeen instances which refer to Jesus keeping the Sabbath.

Basically, the Bible deals with the life stories of God's people and their relationships and experiences with Him. We find that He protects His people, watches over them, and guides them in every situation. It is noted that the people of God are not always obedient; thus, willfully removing themselves from His divine protection.

In the book of Daniel we read of the old prophet being thrown into a den of hungry lions because he was caught praying to God. God protected him through this ordeal and he came forth untouched.

In I Kings we read about the prophet Elijah who became fearful of Jezebel and ran into the wilderness. God sent an angel to bring him food twice a day (I Kings 19:4-8).

God is truly exalted as we read Exodus 14:21-22 which say, "And Moses stretched out his hand over the sea; and the LORD caused the sea to go back by a strong east wind all that night, and the waters were divided. And the children of Israel went into the midst of the sea upon the dry ground: and the waters were a wall unto them on their right hand, and on their left."

In Exodus we were spiritually moved as we read about the children of Israel being led by God through the wilderness. They were led by a pillar of cloud by day and a pillar of fire by night (Exodus 13:21). While they were in the wilderness God rained manna from heaven to feed them. When they murmured (yes, even with all that He had done for them and shown them, they still murmured) He allowed them to eat quails, but He still only fed them two meals a day (Exodus 16:12).

As we continue our search we learn that the fear of God is the beginning of wisdom (Proverbs 9:10) and that knowing the scriptures makes us wise unto salvation (II Timothy 3:15).

All of the scriptures discussed thus far were written by people as they discussed their experiences with God. We looked from Genesis to Revelation and were able to find only one passage which was actually written by God Himself. That passage is *THE TEN COMMANDMENTS (God's Law),* found in Exodus 20:1-17 and repeated in Deuteronomy 5:6-21. Exodus 31:18 tells us that this information was actually written <u>"WITH THE FINGER OF GOD."</u> The Ten Commandment Law is the transcript of God's character. Everything else in the Bible revolves around it.

GOD'S CHARACTER REVEALED

■   God is Love

The major component of God's character (as reflected in The Ten Commandments) is love. If we understand this, we will first love God, then ourselves, then each other.

> "He that loveth not knoweth not God; for God is love."
> I John 4:8

> "And we have known and believed the love that God hath to us. God is love; and he that dwelleth in love dwelleth in God, and God in him."
> I John 4:16

"Love worketh no ill to his neighbour: therefore love is the fulfilling of the law."
Romans 13:10

EXPLORING THE TEN COMMANDMENTS

The very first Commandment of the ten tells us that we must love the God who created: the heavens, the earth, and us, so much that we can have no other god before Him. It is only then that we can love ourselves and our fellow human beings. The first four Commandments teach us how to express our love for God. The last six teach us how to express our love for our fellowmen. Let us explore the Ten Commandments.

THE FIRST FOUR COMMANDMENTS

1. Thou shalt have no other gods before me.

2. Thou shalt not make unto thee any graven image, or any likeness of any thing that is in heaven above, or that is in the earth beneath, or that is in the water under the earth:
Thou shalt not bow down thyself to them, nor serve them: for I the LORD thy God am a jealous God, visiting the iniquity of the fathers upon the children unto the third and

fourth generation of them that hate me;
And Shewing mercy unto thousands of them
that love me, and keep my commandments.
Exodus 20:3-6

We will pause for a moment to point out one of the many scriptures which demonstrate that Jesus Christ of The New Testament is one with the God of the Old Testament. Look at the last sentence of the scripture above and compare it to the one listed below. The words listed below are a direct quote from Jesus Christ.

"If ye love me, keep my
commandments."
John 14:15

3. Thou shalt not take the name of the Lord
thy God in vain; for the Lord will not hold
him guiltless that taketh his name in vain.

Again we pause to highlight a special point. The word "vain" means "useless or without real significance". This scripture lets us know that if we refer to ourselves as children of God; yet, we are not willing to do all that God says, we have taken His name in "vain". This is sin.

4. Remember the sabbath day, to keep it
holy.
Six days shalt thou labour, and do all thy
work:

But the seventh day is the sabbath of the Lord thy God: in it thou shalt not do any work, thou, nor thy son, nor thy daughter, thy manservant, nor thy maidservant, nor thy cattle, nor thy stranger that is within thy gates:

For in six days the Lord made heaven and earth, the sea, and all that in them is, and rested the seventh day: wherefore the Lord blessed the sabbath day, and hallowed it.
Exodus 20:8-11

THE LAST SIX COMMANDMENTS

The last six commandments teach us how to demonstrate our love for each other.

5. Honor thy father and thy mother: that thy days may be long upon the land which the Lord thy God giveth thee.

6. Thou shalt not kill.
Exodus 20:12-13

Again we will pause to highlight a special point. The commandment to not kill includes all types of killing. If we force upon ourselves an early death by not following God's health laws, we are breaking this commandment.

7. Thou shalt not commit adultery.

8. Thou shalt not steal.

9. Thou shalt not bear false witness against thy neighbour.

10. Thou shalt not covet thy neighbour's house, thou shalt not covet thy neighbour's wife, nor his manservant, nor his maidservant, nor his ox, nor his ass, nor any thing that is thy neighbour's.
Exodus 20:14-17

God's health law, like His Ten Commandment Law will exemplify His love.

■   God does not change; therefore, the Ten Commandments and the health laws are unchanging. God's health laws, like His Ten Commandments and His character, will be the same as they have been since the beginning.

"For I am the LORD, I change not; therefore ye sons of Jacob are not consumed."
Malachi 3:6

THE TEN COMMANDMENTS: IN EXISTENCE BEFORE THE CREATION OF PLANET EARTH

The Ten Commandments were written on two tables of stone by God Himself and handed to Moses on Mt. Sinai in 1491 B.C. But, it is a fact that this all important law actually existed before the world was created, (see I John 3:4). It is obvious that these laws existed before Moses' experience on Mt. Sinai because the scriptures tell us that "Sin is the transgression of the law and **WHERE THERE IS NO LAW THERE IS NO SIN**" (Romans 4:5; 5:13).

Lucifer sinned in heaven before the foundation of the world. Iniquity was found in him. He sought to cast his throne above the God of the Most High. He wanted to be God and not be subject to the Godhead (Isaiah 14:12-14). Had there been no law that said, "Thou shalt have no other god before me", and "Thou shalt not covet", disregarding God would not have been a sin.

Satan communicated with Adam and Eve in the Garden of Eden in 4004 B.C. This was almost 2000 years before Moses was born. Satan told the first lie that was told on earth when he said to Eve, "Ye shalt not surely die". Had there been no commandment that said, "Thou shalt not bear false witness", it would have been okay for Satan to tell this lie (Genesis 3:4).

When Eve first, then Adam, disobeyed God's instructions, they became Satan's servants of sin instead of God's innocent, obedient children. To whom you yield yourself servants to obey, his servants you are (see Romans 6:16). Had there been no commandment which said,

"Thou shalt have no other gods before me", this would not have been a problem.

Cain slew his brother Abel almost two thousand years before Moses received the Commandments on Mt. Sinai. If there had been no law which said, "Thou shalt not kill", at this time, it would have been fine for Cain to kill his brother (Genesis 4:8).

In 1729 B.C., Joseph was thrown into prison for refusing to yield to the advances of Potiphar's wife to enter into an adulterous affair with her. This was approximately 300 hundred years before Moses was handed the Ten Commandments on two tables of stone on Mount Sinai. Yet, when she approached him, Joseph said, "How then can I do this great wickedness and sin against God?". If there had been no law already in effect which said, "Thou shalt not commit adultery", Joseph could have avoided a lot of pain and suffering and yielded to her advances and not have had to concern himself about sinning against God (Genesis 39:7-20).

We could have included every situation from Genesis and other parts of the Bible which demonstrate beyond a doubt that God's Ten Commandments were in effect long before it was given to Moses on two tablets of stone on Mount Sinai, but we think you get the picture. This bit of information is contrary to popular belief because most people think that the Ten Commandments were not in existence until they were given to Moses on Mt. Sinai in 1491 B.C. and were changed or totally eradicated in the New Testament with the first coming of Jesus Christ. Look at this scripture quoting Jesus concerning the law of God.

> "Think not that I am come to
> destroy the law, or the
> prophets: I am not come to
> destroy but to fulfil.
> For verily I say unto you, Till
> heaven and earth pass, one jot
> or one tittle shall in no wise
> pass from the law till all be
> fulfilled."
> Matthew 5:17-18

■ God has a definite concern about how we live our lives. He demonstrated this concern by giving us the Ten Commandments to teach us what He wants us to do. In the same sense He has a definite concern about our health and well-being. So, surely He has given us health laws that we need to follow.

> "Beloved, I wish above all
> things that thou mayest
> prosper and be in health, even
> as thy soul prospereth."
> 3 John 2

■ God is a God of order; meaning that He has designed the universe in a specific manner and He has specific instructions for us to follow concerning all things. Just as we have specific Commandments pertaining to our moral lives, we have specific statues related to how to treat our physical bodies.

"Let all things be done decently
and in order."
I Corinthians 14:40

"And said, If thou wilt
diligently hearken to the voice
of the LORD thy God and wilt
do that which is right in his
sight, and wilt give ear to his
commandments, and keep all of
his statues, I will put none of
these diseases upon thee,
which I have brought upon the
Egyptians: for I am the LORD
that healeth thee."
Exodus 15:26

This scripture is proof beyond question that God really does have statues of health and that these statues have far-reaching consequences and are capable of not only maintaining but restoring *GOOD HEALTH.*

■　　God is "no respecter of persons". The Ten Commandments were given to the world, not just to one group of people. The same is true of His Health Laws. Therefore provisions will be made to make the Health Laws simple and available to all regardless of social and economic status or geographic location. They will be accessible to the poor as well as to the rich.

"Then Peter opened his mouth
and said, Of a truth I perceive
that God is no respecter of
persons:"
Acts 10:34

"And when ye reap the harvest
of your land, thou shalt not
wholly reap the corners of thy
field, neither shalt thou gather
the gleanings of thy harvest.
And thou shalt not glean thy
vineyard, neither thou shalt
gather every grape of thy
vineyard; thou shalt leave them
for the poor and stranger: I am
the LORD your God."
Leviticus 19:9,10

If the scriptures above (Leviticus 19:9,10) were
followed as God directed, there would be no hungry people
in the world today.

■   God's Commandments are simple to understand and
easy to follow if we want to follow them. The same
thing will apply to the health laws. They will be
simple to follow and easy to understand.

"For the wisdom of this world is foolishness with God. For it is written, He taketh the wise in their own craftiness."
I Corinthians 3:19

God's health laws, just as the Ten Commandments (the transcript of His character) exemplify love. They are steadfast and do not change. They are orderly and necessary for us to make it through this journey on planet earth. God expects all of us to follow them. He has made them simple to understand; so, we are without excuse (Romans 1:19-20).

Now that we have a basic description of God's character, we have standards by which the Health Laws can be tested.

LEG 13

A THOROUGH SEARCH OF THE BIBLICAL HEALTH LAWS

G OD is a God of order, not chaos. Therefore, He has given the universe, and everything in it a specific design. He has placed all things under rules, regulations, and guidelines; or, under "laws", the popular Biblical term. The Hebrew term "torah" is translated in English as "law". In the Bible, "law", refers to "divine instruction" or revelation from God. There are five Biblical

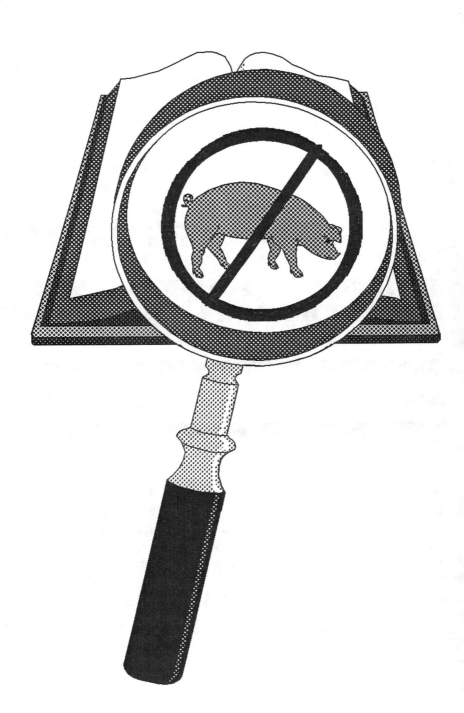

"laws" which are easily identifiable. These laws provide instructions about everything that we need to know in this life.

THE LAWS ARE:

■ **The Natural Law** - which deals with the activities of nature. This law was activated on planet earth "In the beginning" when the Godhead created the heaven and the earth. The sun, moon, and stars are all directed by the natural law. The movement of time and the change from night to day occur through the natural law that God has set forth. A very well known part of the natural law is the law of gravity.

■ **The Civil Law** - which deals with the definite, specific instructions that God has provided to show us how to deal with people in all relationships: husband-wife, parents-children, neighbors-neighbors, worker-employer, and even how we should deal with strangers. This information is primarily found in Leviticus, Exodus, and Corinthians. The many references to the "gate" in the Old Testament deal with legal matters which are a part of the civil law.

■ **The Moral Law** - or the Law of Liberty which is the **TEN COMMANDMENT LAW.** This "perfect" law existed in heaven before the creation of the earth. Most people believe that it was first established on Mt. Sinai when it was presented to Moses on two tables of stone. Actually, the presentation on Mt. Sinai was a reminder to the Children of Israel that they had repeatedly broken God's law. This perfect, unchangeable law was explored thoroughly in Leg 12 of our journey.

■   **The Ceremonial Law** - or SACRIFICIAL LAW which provides definite instructions concerning God's relationship to His people, and the great sacrifice that God makes to redeem them. The scriptures tell us that the "wages of sin is death" (Romans 6:23). Once man succumbed to the evils of sin, there was no alternative other than eternal death. God, in is infinite wisdom and great love, put forth His plan of salvation. In this plan, God Himself would die and suffer the eternal or second death for condemned man. Naturally, God, being God, was totally innocent of any wrong doing.

In the Old Testament man waited for God (the Messiah) to come to earth and die for the sins of man that man might live. Prior to His coming, some people performed certain rituals as a reminder that the Messiah was to come and make this great sacrifice. In some cases these reminders involved sacrificing an innocent animal, usually a lamb, on a regular basis. It pointed toward the coming of the "Messiah".

The New Testament bears witness to the fact that the Messiah, Jesus Christ, came forth. He died for the sins of man. Today, as in the Old Testament, the real requirements of the sacrifice involve "the sacrifice" of living a sin-free life (see Psalms 51:16-19 and Romans 12:1-2).

Partaking of Holy Communion and being baptized are the outward signs that we have accepted Christ and are living free from sin. These ceremonies are practiced today by Christians everywhere to point back to the great sacrifice that Christ made on the cross at Calvary.

■ **The Health Law** - which is where we want to focus our attention because we are *IN SEARCH OF THOSE ACTIVITIES WHICH, WHEN PERFORMED, MAKE HEALTHY BLOOD.* Just as God created everything else in the universe with a specific design and to be governed by specific principles and laws, so He did with the **human being**. The human being is electrical and chemical and has three major components:

■ *The Spiritual Component*

■ *The Mental Component*

■ *The Physical Component*

Each component of the human system has five requirements which must be fulfilled for the system to remain in good health and work properly. The requirements are:

■   *to receive nourishment.*

■   *to indulge in exercise*

■   *to obtain the proper amount of rest and relaxation.*

■   *to have a method of eliminating waste.*

■   *to abstain from injurious substances or elements.*

The Health laws (principles or statues) were put into effect to fulfill the requirements of the system.

In His infinite wisdom and magnificent love, God has given us a certain amount of control over our fate and the status of our health and well-being. He has given us the opportunity to learn of and to follow His health laws. Yet, we are equally free to totally disregard them and do as we please.

Even though we don't have complete control, we can actually **influence** the type diseases that we get. Sometimes, we make the decision of whether or not we recover or succumb to those diseases. Also, we can decide how rapidly we will recover from those diseases or how soon we will succumb to them. These factors are determined by how closely we follow God's health laws.

"The law of the LORD is perfect, converting the soul: the testimony of the LORD is sure, making wise the simple. The statues of the LORD are right, rejoicing the heart: the

commandment of the LORD is pure, enlightening the eyes.
The fear of the LORD is clean, enduring for ever: the judgements of the LORD are true and righteous altogether.
More to be desired are they than gold, yea, than much fine gold: sweeter also than honey and the honeycomb.
Moreover by them is thy servant warned: and in keeping them there is great reward."
Psalm 19:7-11

INTRODUCTION TO GOD'S HEALTH LAWS

In keeping God's Health Laws there, indeed, is great reward. As we explore these laws we will check to see if His character is exemplified in them.

The Health Laws will:

- exemplify love. They will not be harsh or unbearable.

- be orderly and demonstrate God's concern for our health.

- remain unchanged from ancient times to the present.

■   be equally available to all. Health Law #3 deals with the proper diet. Some could make the point that a proper diet is not available to people who are extremely poor. We must look at the fact that if the instructions given in Leviticus 19:9-10 and Matthew 25:31-46 were followed, there would be no people who were too poor to afford a proper diet. Remember, the fact that there are starving people among us, is a result of people **"NOT FOLLOWING"** all OF God's instructions. The problem is not with God or the Health Laws but with people.

■   be simple to understand and follow if there is a desire to do so.

GOD'S HEALTH LAWS

1. LAW: DEEP BREATHING

A.   REFERENCE SCRIPTURE(S)

> "And the *LORD* God formed man of the dust of the ground, and breathed into his nostrils the breath of life and man became a living soul."
> Genesis 2:7

B.   RATIONALE

Deep breathing provides the blood with the much-needed oxygen to be transported to the cells. It moves fresh air in and CO_2 out. The lack of oxygen is much more of a threat to life than the prolonged lack of food or water. Cells must be constantly supplied with oxygen and other nutrients in order to survive and function properly.

Deep breathing strengthens the abdominal muscles so that; eventually, they will begin to rise automatically. This will increase the total amount of air which is moved in and out during regular respirations. With deep breathing, the body is able to move CO_2 and other waste materials out of the system at a much more rapid rate.

C.   SUGGESTED METHOD(S) OF PRACTICE

PROCEDURE # 1.

First of all let us clarify the fact that regular breathing is not *DEEP BREATHING*. Deep breathing exercises should be performed several times a day. Start in the morning prior to performing the regular stretch exercises and do as suggested below.

■   Stand on the floor with the feet approximately six inches apart.

■   Bring both hands to the front and allow the backs of the hands to touch gently.

■ While inhaling (breathing in) slowly, keeping the hands together as they gradually move upward. Flare the nostrils while breathing in.

■ When the hands reach the nose, slowly begin to exhale, (pushing air out). Purse your lips while exhaling.

■ Gradually separate the hands and bring them to a stretched-out shoulder level position.

■ Repeat this procedure at least five times each exercise session.

PROCEDURE #2

■ A second deep-breathing exercise procedure involves lying flat on the back with a small book (only heavy enough to feel its weight) over the abdomen. Breathe deeply enough to make the book rise. As you exhale the book will be lowered. Repeat this exercise five to ten times per session.

D.   NOTABLE RESULTS

One should notice that when the deep breathing exercises are first started, this process moves air in and out of the system at a much more rapid rate than that to which the system has become accustomed. Some people have reported slight dizziness when they first begin to practice this health measure. The dizziness is not noticed by all. Even when it is noticed, it will last for only a few minutes during the exercise period. After a few days this feeling of dizziness no longer occurs during the exercise sessions.

Some of the more notable benefits of deep breathing are: stimulation of the digestive tract which results in improved appetite and a greater desire for the proper diet, more efficient removal of waste through all exit ports, and more efficient and sounder sleep.

2. *LAW: THE USE OF PLENTY OF WATER*

A. *REFERENCE SCRIPTURE*

> "And a river went out of Eden to water the garden; and from thence it was parted, and became into four heads."
> Genesis 2:10

> "And ye shall serve the *LORD* your God, and he shall bless thy bread, and thy water; and I take sickness away from the midst of thee."
> Exodus 23:25

> "And this shall be his uncleanness in issue: whether

his flesh run with his issue, or
his flesh be stopped from his
issue, it is his uncleanness.
Every bed, where upon he lieth
that hath the issue, is unclean:
and every thing, whereon he
sitteth, shall be unclean.
And whosoever toucheth his
bed shall wash his clothes, and
bathe himself in water, and be
unclean until even."
Leviticus 15:3-5

"And when he that hath an
issue is cleansed of his issue;
then he shall number to
himself seven days for his
cleansing, and wash his
clothes, and bathe his flesh in
running water and shall be
clean."
Leviticus 15:13

"Prove thy servants, I beseech
thee, ten days; and let them
give us pulse to eat, and water
to drink."
Daniel 1:12

B.   RATIONALE:

Two-thirds of the human body is water. Most of the plasma of the blood is composed of water. Water is needed to regulate all of the body processes. It is the method by which nutrients enter the blood stream and it is essential in the maintenance of body temperature. Without water the mucous membranes would not remain moist and soft. The intake of a sufficient amount of water is necessary if waste is to be efficiently and rapidly moved from the system. **When an adequate amount of water is in the body the blood is bathed and purified.**

This precious liquid is not only good for the inside, it is also necessary for the system on the outside. Water is the principle factor in the practice of proper hygiene. The entire surface of the body is a vehicle through which waste material passes. Particles of waste from the internal structures of the body collect on the skin. This, plus the dead cells from the skin surface itself, make it necessary for the body to be washed frequently, preferably in running water.

Water is the most appropriate substance available for drinking and cleaning (clothing, people, and the surfaces of objects that must be handled by people).

C.   SUGGESTED METHOD(S) OF PRACTICE

INTERNAL CLEANSING is a major health principle. In order to accomplish this, one should drink six to eight glasses of water each day.

Water should **NOT** be taken with meals.   When water is taken with meals it dilutes the digestive enzymes, and lowers the temperature of the stomach to a level which is not high enough for proper digestion to take place. Food then remains in the stomach too long. The water must, therefore, be absorbed and the temperature of the stomach must return to normal before proper digestion can occur.

Drink cool (not cold) water approximately one hour before meals. Wait at least one hour after a meal before the next glass of water. Between meals and after the last meal, try to drink water hourly up to about three hours before bedtime.

EXTERNAL CLEANSING/PROPER HYGIENE is also crucial for good health.   Skin surfaces should be washed in running water at least on a daily basis. Yes, showering is better than tub baths.

When clothing which directly touch the skin are removed, they should be washed before being worn again. Clothing pick up dead cells and bacteria from the skin. The bacteria feed on the dead cells and quickly multiply. It is a poor hygienic measure to place these dead cells and bacteria next to the skin a second time.

D.   NOTABLE RESULTS

Using water properly, internally and externally, will result in improved health because filth will be more rapidly removed from the body and the cells will be able to work more efficiently. Therefore, all of the sources of elimination of waste will work more efficiently. Such sources of elimination are the urinary system, the colon, the lungs, and the skin. Be prepared to make more frequent trips to the bathroom.

3.   LAW: PROPER DIET

A.   REFERENCE SCRIPTURE

"And God said, Behold, I have given you every herb bearing seed, which is upon the face of all the earth, and every tree, in the which is the fruit of a tree yielding seed; to you it shall be for meat."
Genesis 1:29

B.   RATIONALE

The cells of the body are constantly breaking down and rebuilding tissue. This is a continuous cycle and the correct products are needed for the cells to perform their duties. The products which are required for the entire system to work properly are found in food: water, carbohydrates, proteins, fats, minerals, vitamins, enzymes, and fiber. These substances provide the system with the much needed energy to work appropriately.

The healthiest diet, *(THE DIET WHICH THE ALL MIGHTY GOD ACTUALLY DESIGNED FOR THE BODY)* is the *VEGETARIAN DIET.* Meat is the flesh of a dead animal. Dead animals, regardless of the circumstances under which they died, carry and breed *FILTH*. It cannot be overstated how important it is to total health to constantly rid the body of waste and filth in a timely manner. We read on page 38 and 39 that when an animal dies, much of the waste, which under regular circumstances would be removed **(STOOL, URINE, AND SWEAT)**, is trapped in the tissues of the deceased. Bacteria in this dead flesh grows at a staggering rate. When the flesh of this deceased animal is eaten, digested, and moved into the human blood stream, all of the filth from this flesh also moves into the blood stream. Sadly, when you eat flesh you are actually eating some of the blood, sweat, urine, and feces of that animal. This happens because all of the filth that would, under regular circumstances, be eliminated becomes trapped in the tissues of the dead animal. The blood, already charged with the responsibility of transporting waste and filth from the cells as rapidly as possible, is now given a double, triple, or even greater duty to perform. Putting the flesh of another animal into the system is the same concept as putting clothes in the washing machine with water and three or four cups of dirt, grit, and grime instead of detergent.

Also, the body is designed to digest and process only two meals a day instead of three—*SORRY ! ! !*

C. SUGGESTED METHOD(S) OF PRACTICE

Train your appetite. Appetite training is similar to any other type of training. Use a step-by-step process which allows the stomach to gradually become accustomed to receiving food at certain times and in certain amounts. *SEVERAL RULES RELATED TO TRAINING THE APPETITE* are listed below.

■   Eat at the same times each day.

■   Eat only two meals a day. These two meals should be eaten early in the day, with the second meal being taken at least four to six hours after the first. If a third meal must be taken (during the period of adjustment) make it a one-item meal such as a fruit, a vegetable, a cup of vegetable soup, or a cup of herbal tea. A third meal, no matter how small, is acceptable only during the training period.

■   Always eat breakfast (unless fasting).   *YES, BREAKFAST REALLY IS THE MOST IMPORTANT MEAL OF THE DAY.* Most of the calories for the day should be taken in at the breakfast meal.

■   Let four to six hours lapse between the end of one meal and the beginning of the next. The stomach needs time to empty itself and rest before being filled again.

■   Eat only one serving of the various food items.

■   Refrain from eating between-meal snacks. Snacking, even on foods that are otherwise considered very healthy, is a No-No. The digestive system is able to process and move "vegetarian food" from the stomach in four to six hours. It takes the system much longer to move flesh meat. If food is placed in the stomach before the system is ready to receive it, the process of digestion is started again too soon; thus, overworking the system.

■   Shop for produce grown in good, natural soil rather than food fertilized with synthetic chemicals. Shop at a health food store or holistic health center which carries "organically" grown produce. This will help to assure that you are getting the proper nutrients from your food.

■   Never take liquids with the meals. If liquids must be taken at mealtime (during the transition period) take no more than four ounces. Liquids dilute the digestive juices and lower the temperature of the stomach below that which is needed for proper digestion.

■   Do not clog your system with empty calories (foods which are void of the nutrients required by the body for its proper functioning). Such foods move too slowly through the digestive system; thus, clogging it up. These foods also contribute to weight gain, irritate mucous linings, damage teeth, overstimulate the pancreas, interfere with the natural food instincts, contribute to a deficiency of calcium and mineral salts, and cause peptic ulcers and myocardial infarctions.

All of the above conditions relate to the cells of the body trying desperately to perform their duties but without the proper tools (nutrients) to do so. A partial list of the foods which contain empty calories and do all of this damage are: refined sugar, white rice, white flour, white enriched bread, white corn meal, and colas and other soft drinks.

- Obtain fat, a nutrient which is very much needed in the diet, from natural vegetarian sources: fruits, vegetables, nuts, and grains.

- Eat at least one raw fruit or vegetable at each meal.

- *NEVER, NEVER, NEVER,* eat at bedtime or have a midnight snack. Food in the stomach during the hours of rest interferes with sound sleep because the body is trying to rest while the stomach is busy trying to work.

- Always stop eating when you are full. Never stuff yourself. The stomach area is designed to accommodate only a limited volume of food at one time. An overstuffed stomach puts undue pressure on the stomach walls and the abdominal muscles, and the enzymes available for digestion. Other organs of the body, especially the brain, are overly taxed by an over-stuffed stomach.

- Take the time to plan your meals. Leave nothing to chance. As you select the items to plan a healthy menu, **FORGET** *THE FOUR BASIC FOOD GROUPS* and *OBSERVE GOD'S GARDEN CODE.* God has coded His garden based on **COLOR, CONSISTENCY,** and **CATEGORY.**

CATEGORY: groups foods as: fruits, vegetables, nuts, grains, legumes, and herbs.

COLOR: refers to all of the colors of the rainbow which are found in the various foods.

CONSISTENCY: refers to the texture, shape, and firmness of the food.

■ Eat a wide variety of food. It has been said that "variety is the spice of life". This holds true for meal planning as well. When making selections for meals, make sure you choose **different** foods based on category, color, and consistency.

EXAMPLE: An apple and a pear are in the same category and they are similar in shape, texture, firmness, and in some cases color. Therefore, you would not choose an apple and a pear for the same meal. In the same sense, you should not choose pinto beans and great northern beans, nor should you choose yellow corn and yellow squash for the same meal.

Although, you should choose only three or four food items for each meal, you should be careful to eat a wide variety of foods over a given period of time. Get into the habit of never eating the same food for two meals in a row or for two days in a row. Leftovers should be frozen for a later time or thrown out.

■   When training is over, continue all of the practices listed. You will know that the training is completed when following the listed principles becomes automatic. You will no longer have a desire to practice unhealthy habits.

A SIMPLE MENU PLAN

PRE-BREAKFAST CLEANSER

Herbal tea with one teaspoon of honey and one teaspoon of lemon juice is an excellent cleanser. Have this drink each morning and then wait approximately one hour before having breakfast.

A GENEROUS BREAKFAST

THIS IS GOING TO SEEM STRANGE, BUT......

A generous breakfast should consist of what you would probably have for lunch or dinner.

Three Vegetables (at least one should be raw)

One serving of Whole Grain Bread

No Liquid for at least one hour

OR IF YOU INSIST ON TRADITION

A Whole Grain Cereal

Two Fruits (one or both should be raw)

One serving of Whole Grain Bread

No Liquid for at least one hour

A LIBERAL LUNCH

A Whole Grain Cereal

Two Fruits (one or both should be raw)

One serving of Whole Grain Bread

> **OR**
>
> No Liquid for at least one hour
>
> Two or three Vegetables
>
> One serving of Whole Grain Bread

A LIGHT OR NON-EXISTENT SUPPER

Basically, we should omit the third meal. If, during the training period, an evening meal is required, it should consist of only one item.

> One small vegetable,
>
> **OR**
>
> One small fruit,
>
> **OR**
>
> A small bowl of vegetable soup,
>
> **OR**
>
> One small salad,
>
> **OR**
>
> A cup of herbal tea.

GENERAL INSTRUCTIONS RELATED TO MEALS

Let water be your between-meal snack. Allow one hour to lapse between breakfast and the first glass of water. Continue drinking water, (one glass every hour, approximately six to eight ounces per glass) until a total of six to eight glasses have been consumed for the day. Be careful to assure that the last meal is consumed at least four to six hours before bedtime. The last glass of water should be consumed no closer than three hours before bedtime.

If you are thinking, "It is impossible for me to drink six to eight ounces of water at one time", then try three or four ounces. As your system becomes trained, it will be able to tolerate more. All people do not require the exact same amount of water.

D.   *NOTABLE RESULTS*

Bowel movements will begin to occur at least once or twice a day, usually after each meal. The amount of waste material evacuated from the body through the bowel will markedly increase. If there was a problem with constipation, it will disappear.

Though the volume of the stool is greater, the time spent moving the bowels will dramatically decrease. All of the waste will be delivered from the body effortlessly and almost in an instant.

The stools will weigh a lot less. Typically when flesh is included in the diet, the stools will weigh about two or three pounds. When people who eat flesh begin a reduction diet, they like to weigh after a bowel movement because they will weigh two to three pounds less. The stools of a vegetarian, even though more massive, will usually weigh less than a pound. Unless your system has lost a measurable amount of fluid, it won't help much to wait until after a bowel movement to weigh.

Another very dramatic change that you will notice is the change in the odor of the stools. Believe it or not, the stools become almost odorless. There is a very slight odor but it is not a pungent, foul smell as before.

E. A NOTABLE CONCERN

When people who have typically included flesh meat in the diet become vegetarians; frequently, they will notice an increase in abdominal discomfort due to "gas". This problem will go away after a while but can be very uncomfortable while it lasts. Many health food stores will carry a digestive enzyme which will provide a great deal of relief. Once all of the digestive enzyme has been taken, the system will have adjusted to its new life style and the discomfort will be gone.

4. LAW: PERIODIC FASTING

A. REFERENCE SCRIPTURE

"Is not this the fast that I have chosen? to loose the bands of wickedness, to undo the heavy burdens, and to let the oppressed go free, and that ye break every yoke?

Is it not to deal thy bread to the hungry, and that thou bring the poor that are cast out to thy house? when thou seest the naked, that thou cover him; and that thou hide not thyself from thine own flesh?

Then shall thy light break forth as the morning, and thine health shall spring forth speedily: and thy righteousness shall go before thee; the glory of the LORD shall be thy rereward."

Isaiah 58:6-8

"And Jesus said unto them, Because of your unbelief: for verily I say unto you, if ye have faith as a grain of mustard seed, ye shall say unto this mountain, Remove hence to yonder place; and it shall remove; and nothing shall be impossible unto you.

Howbeit this kind goeth not out but by prayer and fasting."

Matthew 17:20-21

B.   RATIONALE

When we look up the word "fast", we learn that it is a homonym. It has many meanings such as: to move quickly or rapidly; extreme energy; resistant, such as acid-fast; or firmly fixed, as in unmovable; and deep or sound, as in fast asleep. All of these definitions can apply when we "fast" to improve our health. We move rapidly to a state of improved health and we become more soundly and firmly fixed in our spiritual relationship with God.

Fasting simply refers to abstinence from something, in most cases food; but it can pertain to abstinence from anything. During a food fast one should select certain foods to omit from the diet for a specified period of time.

Fasting falls into the following categories:

- a selected item fast - such items as: sweets or flesh meats, etc. are removed from the diet for a period of time.

- a liquid or juice fast - when only vegetable or fruit juices are taken for a period of time.

- a water fast - only water is taken into the body during the fasting period.

- the total fast - nothing is taken by mouth, (not even water) for a period of time.

■   the true fast - when every undesirable act is removed from the life's activities throughout existence. All Christians should strive for the true fast.

Throughout Biblical history, fasting from food has been used as a method of gaining spiritual strength. In most cases the actual period of the fast was varied. There are examples of periods of fasting from one evening to forty days.

In 510 B.C., the Jews were threatened with annihilation by Haman. Esther was asked by Mordecai to make supplication unto the king on behalf of the Jews. At first, Esther was reluctant, but was urged on by Mordecai ("Who knoweth whether thou art come to the kingdom for such a time as this?", Esther 4:14). Esther requested that all of the Jews and her maidens fast ("neither eat nor drink for three days"). The Jews received the victory and Haman was executed on his own gallows.

In 27 A.D. Jesus fasted forty days and forty nights. He had just been baptized and was preparing to start His ministry. Christians know and love Jesus as a member of the Godhead and as the greatest teacher and religious leader that the world has ever known.

SHORT PERIODIC FASTS

Short (three days or less), periodic fasts are very beneficial physically, mentally, and spiritually.

Physically, fasting accelerates the removal of waste material from all exit ports of the body. This is a very healthy procedure in itself, but the greatest physical benefit lies in the fact that while fasting, the body actually breaks down and removes damaged and diseased cells from the system.

Mentally, we become more alert; and spiritually, we are able to get closer to our Lord and Savior.

Short periods of fasting can be used as a very efficient method of gaining the victory over appetite and other harmful habits.

When a longer fast is chosen, we must remember that it takes a special procedure to start and end the fast in a healthy manner.

However, we need to keep in mind the fact that we are not required by God to go on long fasts in order to get closer to Him, nor is it a health requirement. God is interested in us: loving Him, ourselves, each other, and in our following all of His commandments.

C.   SUGGESTED METHOD(S) OF PRACTICE

SHORT FASTS

Very short fasts involve one to three days or one or two meals. Just pick a period of time to omit certain things or all things from the diet. It is not a good idea to omit everything (including water) from the diet for more than a day. If you choose a very short fast and decide to just eliminate a meal, always choose to fast the last meal of the day. Never choose to eliminate breakfast.

LONG FASTS
PREPARATION

STEP ONE (PREPARATION)

Eliminate from the diet all flesh meats, dairy products, soft drinks, and any foods classified as junk food or foods containing empty calories. Follow the diet plan on page 139-141 for several days.

STEP TWO

Eliminate nuts and grains from the diet. Use herbal tea for the pre-breakfast cleansing. For breakfast, consume a variety of raw fruits. For lunch, eat a garden salad with fresh lemon juice as the salad dressing. Drink water every hour between meals.

THE ACTUAL FAST

DAY ONE

Eliminate all solid food. Drink only herbal tea and **RAW** fruit and vegetable **juices.** These juices can be obtained from a health food store or with the use of a juicer. Raw juice should be mixed half and half with water. Drink the raw juice whenever you feel hungry. These juices can be mixed, (traditional fruits with traditional fruits and traditional vegetables with traditional vegetables). Do not mix fruit juices with vegetable juices.

DAY TWO

Repeat day one of the actual fast.

DAY THREE

Repeat day one of the actual fast (if desired).

DAY FOUR

Repeat day one of the actual fast (if desired).

DAY FIVE (BREAKING THE FAST)

Add a raw fruit salad for breakfast and a raw vegetable salad for lunch. Continue the juices.

DAY SIX

Add one cooked food item for each of the two meals; something such as a baked potato, stewed prunes, or a baked apple.

DAY SEVEN

The same as day six. Add a bowl of homemade soup.

DAY EIGHT

Begin using the Proper Diet plan listed on page 139-141 and continue throughout this earthly life. Vegetarians can start a fast beginning with step two.

D.   NOTABLE RESULTS

The texture of the skin and hair will change and take on a silky appearance. The frequency of urination will increase dramatically. After the fast, your whole system will feel clean and light. You will feel closer to God and more able to accomplish difficult tasks.

One change which may be considered strange will occur. All other health measures cause the body odor to all but disappear. This one health principle will cause the body--especially the breath, to have a foul odor. This foul odor occurs because diseased tissue is being broken down and removed from the system. Once the fasting period is completed, the system is again rendered practically odor free. Just as it is with every other problem or concern, vegetarians have less of a problem with odor while fasting than flesh eaters.

5. LAW: GET PLENTY OF SUNSHINE

A. REFERENCE SCRIPTURE(S)

> "And God said, Let there be light: and there was light. And God saw the light, that it was good: and God divided the light from the darkness."
> Genesis 1:3-4

> "Truly the light is sweet, and a pleasant thing it is for the eyes to behold the sun:"
> Ecclesiastes 11:7

B. RATIONALE

The sun is the most powerful (external) healing agent that God has provided. The light from the sun does all of the following:

■   sterilizes the air and articles.

■   enhances the flow of blood to the tissues.

■   restores energy.

■   synthesizes vitamin D.

■   soothes the nervous system.

C.   SUGGESTED METHOD(S) OF PRACTICE

Indulge in activities such as walking, gardening, and simple sports.

Let the sunshine into your home. Open the curtains and allow the sun to especially shine in your kitchen and bedroom. Leave the bed covers pulled back and let the sun shine into your bed.

D.   NOTABLE RESULTS

Benefits will definitely be obtained but they may be difficult to personally detect as separate from the benefits that come as a result of following all of the other health principles. You may, however, notice that your curtains are fading; but, stick with the sunshine, you can always get new curtains but God gave you only one you.

6. LAW: NATURAL EXERCISE

A.   REFERENCE SCRIPTURE(S)

"And the Lord God took the man, and put him into the garden of Eden to dress it and to keep it."
Genesis 2:15

B.   *RATIONALE*

Exercise is simply the act of moving muscles. The benefits of natural exercise comprise a very long list. Natural exercise:

■   enhances the circulation of blood throughout the system.

■   causes the respiratory muscle to develop in strength and capacity.

■   renders the system more resistent to disease and physical disability.

■   assists in the maintenance of good posture.

■   accelerates the movement of waste from the body through all modes of elimination: skin, lungs, kidneys, and the bowel.

■   promotes alertness.

■   eliminates insomnia and promotes sound sleep.

■   neutralizes stress.

■   reduces the negative effects of excessive stress.

C.   SUGGESTED METHOD(S) OF PRACTICE

STRETCH EXERCISES

Stretch exercises prepare the body for more strenuous activity and strengthen and firm muscles. Some simple stretch exercises are:

■   Deep breathing: (see pages <u>127 & 128</u>)

■   Toe touch: stand with your feet approximately 6 inches apart. Bend from the waist forward to touch your toes.

■   Side bends: stand with your feet approximately 6 inches apart. Bend from the waist to the side.

■   Knee bends: stand with your feet together, bend your knees to a sitting position.

■   Leg lifts: lie flat on your back and keep your legs straight. Slowly lift your legs (together) a few inches from the floor. Hold this position for a certain amount of time which will be progressively increased.

These exercises should be started at a slow pace and progressively increased. If you have been basically sedentary or are overweight, you should start with no more than four or six repetitions. Every three or four days increase the number of repetitions by two until you are able to perform between 20 or 30 per exercise session. Go even higher if your system can tolerate it.

SIMPLE AEROBIC EXERCISES

Don't get upset, you won't have to indulge in cross-country skiing, or parachuting. One of the best, easiest, cheapest, and most available aerobic exercises is brisk walking.

People who are usually sedentary should not start an exercise program rapidly--even with something as simple as walking.

Start your program by finding and measuring several specific, scenic routes. Never limit yourself to one route. If you plan to walk through your neighborhood, **drive** through the areas first. Identify points on the routes to mark off certain distances. Watch the speedometer on your car and mark off 1/2 mile, 1 mile, and 1 1/2 mile points up to five miles. Write down street names, addresses; or other specific land marks such as trees, buildings, etc., to let you know when you have reached certain distances.

Start slowly, walk for short periods of time each day and gradually increase the time and distance of the walk. If you do not already have an exercise program, start by walking for about 15 to 20 minutes each day. Record the distance that you have walked. After three or four days, increase the distance by one-half mile every three or four days. Gradually increase the distance until you are walking about four or five miles a day. If you can walk this stretch in 45 minutes to one hour, you are doing very good.

People who are already very active in excess of this amount need not slow down or change their pace in any way. Walking down steps and hills can provide several times the benefit of walking on flat surfaces. Walking up hills and steps can afford up to ten times the benefit of walking on flat surfaces.

D.   NOTABLE RESULTS

The first thing that you will probably notice is sore muscles, but don't despair, this is why you start slowly. After a few days the soreness will go away. Within a few days to a week, you will notice:

■   an increase in your energy levels.

■   sounder sleep.

■   softer, smoother, moister, more viable skin.

■   an improved ability to breath deeply.

SPECIAL NOTE

If you are overweight when you begin keeping all of God's Health Laws, it may take longer for you to notice an increase in your energy level. Your body will gradually begin the process of bringing itself to its correct weight. Reducing fat and building muscle tissue takes a lot of energy. Usually, you will not have less energy than when you began your plan, it may just take longer for you to notice the increase in energy.

7. LAW: REST, RELAXATION, SLEEP

A. REFERENCE SCRIPTURE(S)

"Thus the heavens and the earth were finished, and all the host of them.
And on the seventh day God ended his work which He had made; and He rested on the seventh day from all his work which He had made."
Genesis 2:1-2

"And he lighted upon a certain place, and tarried there all night, because the sun was set; and he took of the stones of that place, and put them for his pillows, and lay down in that place to sleep."
Genesis 28:11

B. RATIONALE

Rest, relaxation, and sleep all represent periods of time in which an individual changes course, moving from a state of activity to a state of suspension of or a change of activity.

Sometimes the terms sleep, rest, and relaxation are used interchangeably, but for our purposes, we will distinguish between the three.

1.   *REST:*   short periodic breaks from regular activities. If you walk up a flight of stairs, you may choose to stop and REST before going up the second flight. Or, upon finishing one project at work, you may choose to REST a few minutes before starting on the next one.

Rest also includes longer periods of time. It is a good idea to set aside at least one twenty-four hour period in each week as a period of rest. During this period, we should not indulge in the exact same activities that are a part of our routine activities for the other days of the week. After creating the world in six days, God rested on the seventh day. He did not go to sleep, He ceased from the activities that He had performed all week.

2.   *RELAXATION:*   basically refers to that state when the muscles of the body move from a state of tension to a state

of ease or release from the tenseness. Sitting in a quiet space and practicing slow, deep breathing can initiate a period of relaxation.

3.   *SLEEP:*   a physiological state of inactivity in which one becomes unaware of the external environment. As we move through our busy schedules, performing all of the activities required for us to make it through the day, a great deal of stress and "wear and tear" is placed upon our bodies. The healing of our tired, worn bodies actually takes place during sleep. This is when the body rebuilds tissues and revitalizes itself; thus, making sleep an essential element in the healing process. During this period the nerves are also soothed and stress is relieved.

C.   SUGGESTED METHOD(S) OF PRACTICE

REST: Follow the example set forth by the creator and designer of the universe. Honor the weekly seventh-day Sabbath. Rest this one day of the week by stopping all of the activities that have been followed all week.

RELAXATION: Train your muscles to be able to recognize the difference between tension and relaxation. During the stretch exercises, note this difference. When periods of stress occur, move the body to a state of relaxation by remembering how the muscles feel when they are relaxed.

SLEEP: Eight hours has been set as the standard amount of sleep required in a 24-hour period. Yet, eight hours can be looked upon as a minimum amount of sleep needed and not a maximum. In God's infinite wisdom and great plan for our optimum health, He made the darkness for sleep and the light for us to carry on our activities. So it follows, since darkness usually lasts longer than eight hours, the body's requirement for sleep is likely more than eight hours. Also, since the hours of darkness are longer in the wintertime than in the summertime, the body requires more sleep in the wintertime. You may have already made up your mind that you cannot or will not sleep from sunset to sunrise, but at the same time, make a point to never begrudge yourself a few extra hours sleep if you need them or when you feel especially tired.

It is essential that sleep be obtained without interference. All of the following things interfere with good sound sleep: **noise, night lights, unrelieved tension, worry about the concerns of the past day, worry about the concerns of tomorrow; a full stomach, and toxins which irritate and stimulate the nervous system; such as caffeine**

or nicotine. It is often that people are heard to say such things as, "I can't sleep without a night light" or "I must have the radio or the TV on before I can go to sleep". In such cases, we have convinced ourselves that these things are necessary for us to sleep soundly when actually they rob us of our proper sleep.

In order for us to gain the most from our period of sleep, several things are important for us to remember. We should:

■   try to reach total darkness. Turn off inside night lights and hall lights. The light coming in from the street should be blocked as much as possible.

■   seek total quietness. Trains, planes, honking car horns, croaking frogs, and barking dogs all interfere with a good night's sleep.

■   go to bed when you feel tired or sleepy. Don't force yourself to stay up to finish a project or to watch a movie.

■   stick to your daily cut off periods for food and drink so that the digestive system will not be trying to work while the rest of the body is trying to sleep.

■   stop worrying and thank God for watching over you the entire day and trust that He will care for you during the night and the following day.

D.   NOTABLE RESULTS

In a short period of time you will notice a feeling of greater peace and contentment. Incidents which once stimulated a great deal of distress are now much less irritating.

8. LAW: TEMPERANCE

A.   REFERENCE SCRIPTURE(S)

"But the fruit of the spirit is love, joy, peace, longsuffering, gentleness, goodness, faith, meekness, temperance: against such there is no law."
Galatians 5:22,23

B.   RATIONALE

Temperance is the practice of:

- abstaining from all injurious substances.

- taking or using all substances that are classified as "good for us" in moderation.

■   abstaining from all injurious
     activities.

■   performing all activities that
     are classified as "good for us"
     in moderation.

God does all things decently and in order. He designed parts of the universe (the parts which can be comprehended by people) to be electrical and chemical. The human body is also designed to be electrical and chemical. It does not take a doctorate in chemistry to figure out that any chemical in the universe cannot be arbitrarily mixed with any other chemical in the universe in any proportion and positive results be obtained. It logically follows that since the human body is electrical and chemical, there are substances in the environment **WHICH WERE NEVER MEANT** to mix with the chemicals in the human body. And, it logically follows that those substances which **WERE** designed to mix with the human body were designed to be mixed (or used) in certain proportions.

A good analogy for this is to consider your experiences in the high school chemistry lab. Your teacher wanted you to perform some experiments. So he or she gave you a formula or some other type of guide to follow. This guide told you which chemicals to select for the experiment. It also gave you the exact amount of each chemical, the temperature, and exactly when and under which circumstances each ingredient was to be added. Under no circumstances would you have been allowed to just start mixing any chemicals in any amount. The same principles apply to the human body. It behooves us to give serious thought to the substances that God designed the human body to mix with and the amounts and circumstances that He specified for mixing them.

Electrical and chemical substances which were designed to mix with the human body are: water, air, sunshine, and the substances in fruits, nuts, vegetables, grains, legumes, and certain herbs.

Food items should be taken in their "natural states". The term "natural states" does not exclude cooking (although most foods are healthier raw), but it does exclude processed foods. Processing robs foods of their nutritional value.

A partial list of substances which were **NOT** designed to mix with the human body include:

- ■   *CAFFEINE* - a chemical found in coffee, chocolate, colas, many other soft drinks, and many teas. It is a major irritant and stimulant to the nervous system.

- ■   *ALCOHOL* - a central nervous system depressant, is a chemical which uses a tremendous amount of vitamin B for its synthesis. This renders the body nervous and irritable, and can lead to damaged nerve cells.

- ■   *TOBACCO* - in all its forms: cigarettes, cigars, pipe tobacco, snuff, and chewing tobacco, is injurious to the system.

Smoke paralyzes the cilia in the nose. The cilia or hairs in the nose were designed by God to catch certain particles which enter the nose during the inhalation period. The particles are then swept out of the nose during exhalation. When the cilia are paralyzed, poisons from the atmosphere are dumped into the lungs. This is a major factor in many serious diseases such as lung cancer and emphysema.

There are many dangerous substances in tobacco which cause: cancer in all parts of the body, emphysema, and heart disease. Chewing tobacco, snuff, and tobacco in other forms are related to cancer of the mouth.

- *SUGAR* - is an empty calorie, meaning that it contains calories which lead to weight gain but it does not contain sufficient amounts of nutrients to justify its use. Sugar enters the blood stream at a very rapid rate and stimulates the pancreas to over react.

- *CONDIMENTS* - such as pepper, ginger, vinegar, chili, nutmeg, and baking soda all irritate the lining of the stomach; thus, interfering with proper digestion.

- *PROCESSED DE-GERMINATED FOODS* - such as white flour, white bread, white rice, white meal, and white sugar are all foods which have had the nutrients stripped from them. These items are sometimes referred to as the "WHITE PLAGUE". They are the end products of foods which have been altered and are no longer in their natural states. They have been put through a process which removed the fiber, minerals, vitamins, and enzymes. When a **FEW** of these nutrients are replaced, these foods are labeled **ENRICHED.**

■ *FLESH MEAT* - is not fit for human consumption. The human body was designed by God to receive the ingredients needed to make **GOOD HEALTHY BLOOD** from **THE PLANT KINGDOM**. The flesh of another animal is too complex and concentrated to be easily and properly assimilated into the human system. The person who eats meat has the double duty of removing filth accumulated from the work of his/her own cells along with processing and synthesizing the animal's filth. A human being can accomplish this only because the body is fearfully and wonderfully made (see Psalms 139:14).

A second point to consider is the fact that; although, people are able to synthesize this flesh, it is not without a great toll being placed upon the body. Overall, as demonstrated in the scriptures (see: the Bible texts which denote the fact that the human life span has progressively declined, Genesis 1:29, and Daniel chapter 1), and modern research, people who eat meat are less healthy and have a shorter life span than people who are vegetarians.

The second part of the temperance definition deals with the partaking of all things in moderation. The human body was designed to use substances in certain amounts and within certain time frames. Overuse of things (even something good) or neglecting to obtain something which is required results in negative effects upon the system.

The third part of the definition of temperance relates to abstinence from all harmful activities. This means any and all such activities as over-reacting to circumstances, riding in a car with an intoxicated or reckless driver, driving reckless yourself, and exposing yourself to infections by walking in the rain without the proper clothing.

The fourth part of this definition deals with performing all activities which are good for the system in moderation. This includes performing all of the statues of health, but being careful to not "over do it". Some examples are: being a glutton, over-exercising, ad infinitum.

It is a very serious health hazard for sedentary people to begin an exercise program at a very rapid rate.

C.   SUGGESTED METHOD(S) OF PRACTICE

In order to put temperance into practice, it is important for us to **LEARN** as much as we can about our bodies and how they interact with the various substances in the environment. We need to take an active role in the maintenance of our health by **not** indulging in harmful activities and doing all good things in moderation.

D.   NOTABLE RESULTS

The results to be expected are equivalent to the geometrical cumulative effect of all notable results mentioned thus far.

9. LAW: NATURAL HEALING

A.   REFERENCE SCRIPTURE(S)

"And the woman said unto the serpent, We may eat of the fruit of the trees of the garden: But of the fruit of the tree which is in the midst of the garden, God hath said, Ye shall not eat of it, neither shall ye touch it, lest ye die."
Genesis 3:2,3

"He causeth the grass to grow
for the cattle, and herb for the
service of man: that he may
bring forth food out of the
earth;"
Psalm 104:14

"And said, If thou wilt
diligently hearken to the voice
of the LORD thy God, and wilt
do that which is right in his
sight, and wilt give ear to his
commandments, and keep all of
his statues, I will put none of
these diseases upon thee,
which I have brought upon the
Egyptians: for I am the LORD
that healeth thee."
Exodus 15:26

B.   RATIONALE

GOD'S original plan was for people to live forever.
When our original parents turned away from God through
disobedience, they invited death to come creeping into the
world. At the very moment that Adam and Eve bit into the
forbidden fruit, they began to die, a little at a time. From
that fateful day, death has been passed from generation to
generation. Since our systems are dying constantly, it is
always necessary for our systems to rebuild and heal.

Through His marvelous love and infinite wisdom, God has placed the substances which activate His healing power in places that are available to us. His healing power is in our blood and tissues and is activated by the air, water, food, sunshine, and certain activities. The activities listed as laws of health: deep breathing, drinking water at the proper times, eating properly, fasting, exercising, resting, practicing temperance, and positive thinking, promote the natural healing process.

As far as food is concerned, there is one type of food that God has specifically designed to promote the healing process. He actually placed medicinal properties is this food. This food is the **HERBS.** Herbs are special plants which are better known for their seasoning capabilities. Two of the best known and most commonly used herbs are garlic and onions.

For every ailment visited upon mankind, God has given us an herb to deal with it. Herbs and **NOT** medications (sorry, not even prescription or over-the-counter medications) were designed for the healing of our bodies.

Of course, we need to clarify one fact. Medications have a very definite effect upon the body, basically they do what the literature about them says that they will do. But, there are two major problems with medications:

■   The first problem with medications is that they do their jobs almost too dramatically. To understand this more fully, let us suppose that you are tired and decide to take something to help you relax and go to sleep.

There are herbs which are specifically designed for this purpose. They will soothe your nervous system and have the effect of lulling you to sleep. You will wake up the next morning feeling relaxed and well-rested. A sleeping pill will also put you to sleep; but, it could have an effect that is similar to a blow on the head from a hammer. You may wake up the next morning feeling tired and worn out.

■   The second problem with medications is that while they are fixing up one part of the body, they are busy messing-up another part. A close examination of a Physician's Desk Reference (PDR) will quickly convince you of this fact when you read the information listed under the headings, "contraindications", "warnings", "precautions", and "adverse effects".

We know, you are going to make the point that many medications are made from herbs. True, True, we concede. But, when medications are made from herbs, the herbs are no longer in their natural state. The drug companies use concentrations which render the medications many times more potent than the herb is in its natural state.

C.   *SUGGESTED METHOD(S) OF PRACTICE*

Use bell peppers, onions, and garlic to season vegetables. Become acquainted with all of the healing herbs. Go to one of the local book stores or health food stores and purchase a book on herbs.

D.   NOTABLE RESULTS

- improved appetite.

- increased energy.

- more rapid healing of ailments.

- chronic complaints either completely disappear or become less irritating.

10. LAW: MAINTAINING A POSITIVE ATTITUDE

A.   *REFERENCE SCRIPTURE(S)*

> "For as he thinketh in his heart, so is he:"
> Proverbs 23:7

B.   RATIONALE

Attitude, controlled by the spiritual aspect of the human system, refers to a state of mind or a feeling on certain issues.   God designed the human body to be physical, mental, and spiritual.   There must be a proper coordination of the three for total health to exist.

The physical part of the system is the part that is most easily understood.   It is the tangible body composed of its eleven systems.   This is usually where all of the focus is placed.

The mental element is as important as the physical; but, much less easily understood.   It relates to the mind or the intellect.   It is the part of the system in which we know, understand, or comprehend things.

The spiritual part is the component of the human system which is the least understood of the three.   We do know that our belief system resides in the spirit and it is through the spirit that we communicate with our God.   God is a spirit and we must worship Him in spirit and truth.

The body can exist without the mental and spiritual components being active (in such a state the individual is referred to as a vegetable).   But, contrary to popular belief, the spirit does not exist without the body and the mental capacities.

The attitude is a part of the belief system that resides within the spirit.   One can have a negative attitude or a positive attitude.

Examples of a Positive Attitude:

■ God has given me charge and responsibility over certain things in my life.

■ I cannot control everything, but I can control some things.

■ God loved me enough to create me.

■ Sometimes things happen to me that I consider good and at other times things happen to me that I consider bad.

■ No matter what happens, I know that God is still in control of this universe.

■ When things that I consider bad happen, there is a reason. I don't always know the reason, but there is a reason. The event may be to help me grow spiritually or for me to learn something beneficial. It may be to allow me to be a witness for someone else or to perform some special work for Christ. Whatever my circumstances or problems that exist in my life, I know that God loves me and that He is in control. Through His divine guidance, He won't let anything happen to me that He and I won't be able to handle together.

Examples of A Bad Attitude:

- Whatever will happen will happen. I can't control anything. God may be able to control certain things, but He won't. He doesn't care about me anyway.

- There is no God.

- I have to live for today. I will do whatever I want and just hope for the best.

- You have to die with something, so it may as well be with ...

- How do I know if "that" has anything to do with my health anyway.

- I know "____" who smoked without ceasing, drank, and did whatever she/he wanted all of his/her life. She/he never had a sick day in his/her life. I am going to do just like "____".

C.   SUGGESTED METHOD(S) of PRACTICE

- The best way to develop a positive attitude is to surrender your thoughts to Christ. Make this surrender effective by asking Christ to totally control your thoughts.

■   Incorporate a Christian **"Motto"** into your lifestyle. A motto is a short statement or group of words which you allow to become a "state of mind" for you. Mottos are built on certain doctrines or truths and are very powerful. They contain words which can be used as a guide for all aspects of your life.

A favorite motto among Christians is found in Philippians 4:13, "I can do all things through Christ which strengthenth me." Other Christian mottos are: "All that God says, I will do, If I perish (Esther 4:26), I perish"; and "There is nothing that will happen to me today that God and I can't handle".

■   Another tangible thing that can be done to enhance a positive attitude is to develop a Philosophy of Life. A Philosophy of Life is a pledge or a commitment to do certain things. And, as with a motto, it should be based on sound doctrines and truths. The Ten Commandments (Exodus 20:1-17), and The True Fast (Isaiah 58:1-14 and Matthew 25:31-46) are excellent doctrines for developing a Philosophy of Life. These doctrines are the bases of the Health Laws.

D.   NOTABLE RESULTS

A positive attitude is physically, spiritually, and mentally healthy. The truly difficult times in life seem to become few and far-in-between. Things that you once thought were impossible to bear are now seen as minor irritations. You begin to feel better about yourself, your ability to handle certain things, and about the people around you.

A negative attitude drains the system mentally, physically, and spiritually.

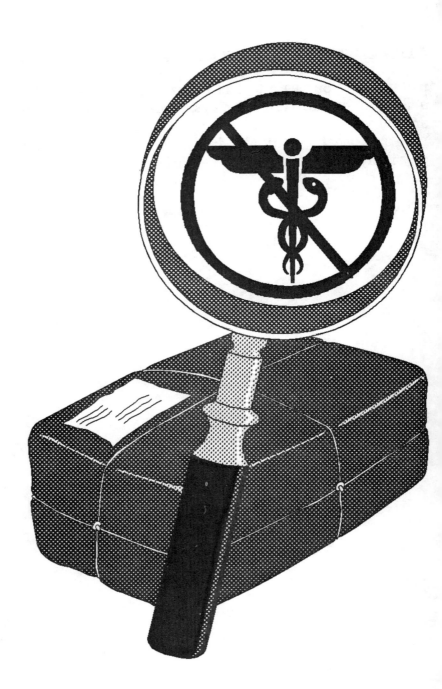

LEG 14

WHAT CAN WE EXPECT FROM FOLLOWING THE HEALTH LAWS?

R ESEARCH informs us that people who follow the principles of health live longer, more productive lives than those who do not. How much longer ? ? . . How much more productive ? ? . . Well, that depends on the number of principles being followed, the status of the uncontrollable health indicators, and who is reporting the research. Though, sometimes the researchers will quote different specific numbers, if we averaged the various numbers, we probably would see that people who follow all of the health laws will live about 6 to 11 years longer than those who do not.

In addition to living longer, people who follow all of the health laws have far fewer diseases and other time, energy, and financially draining conditions.

Rather than concern ourselves with the research, we will devise a plan to determine how much benefit we can detect in ourselves.

Before making changes, make an assessment of your present state of health (see the appendix). Start practicing each health law gradually and progressively and watch for the changes.

The first thing that you may notice is that your body may respond to these changes in a manner that makes you feel slightly ill (see notable results at the end of each section of the health laws). But, keep in mind, this feeling is caused by poisons, which have been embedded in your tissues, being lifted out of your system and the fact that any change is stressful. So, just bear with it; after a few days the ill feelings will go away.

OVERALL NOTABLE CHANGES

WEIGHT - If you are overweight or underweight, your body will gradually begin to move toward the weight that is normal for your height and bone structure.

BOWEL HABITS - Constipation will no longer be a concern. Other digestive problems will be eliminated or greatly reduced.   The stools will actually increase in amount and frequency but will be lighter in weight. Typically, you will begin to move your bowels after each meal and no less than once a day.

SLEEP - You will experience sounder, more beneficial sleep. On most mornings you will be able to wake up on your own, without an alarm clock or wake-up service.

APPEARANCE - Skin problems will be totally eliminated or greatly reduced. The texture of your hair and skin will become softer and more manageable.

VITAL SIGNS/BLOOD VALUES - Your blood pressure, pulse, and respiration will become lower and stronger. Some of the values from blood tests (especially the hematocrit) will become lower. Your test results may become even lower than what is considered "normal". Of course, you do not need to worry about this because, "normal" levels are derived from the tests done on "normal" people. If you go back and review the health laws, you will note that the average or "normal" person does not follow them. Therefore, the "normal" people are not the "healthiest" people.

If you are not following the health laws and all of your vital signs and blood levels are lowered, you probably do have something to worry about.

THE BODY AS A UNIT - your whole body will begin to respond as it is trained.

- You will become hungry, only, just before meal times. You will not have a desire for between-meal or midnight snacks.

- You will notice that you become thirsty when it is time for your water (about an hour after meals and hourly until your next meal or a few hours before bedtime). You will have little or no desire for liquids with your meals.

- Your body will feel like walking at the routine times.

- You will feel sleepy when it is time for you to go to sleep and you will be able to wake up when it is time to start your day.

- You will note that you have more energy.

- Basically, the unnecessary stresses will be removed from your life and you will be more physically, mentally, and spiritually able to deal with the unavoidable stresses that occur. Your temperament will be more relaxed. You may notice that you will be more patient and tolerant of the short comings in others.

- You will catch very few or no colds. If under extenuating circumstances, you do catch a cold, it will be very mild and short in duration.

■ Your thinking will become clearer and you will notice an improved ability to remember things.

■ Your understanding of simple and complex things will be greatly improved.

■ Your body will become more flexible. You will probably notice that you will be able to move faster and more accurately.

■ Minor injuries and bruises will heal much faster.

■ One of the most dramatic changes that you will notice will be the change in the odor of your body, body fluids, and body waste. Perspiration, even after strenuous exercise, will be practically odorless. Also, there will be no stringent foul odor when you go to the bathroom. Your urine and even stool will be virtually odorless unless you are fasting.

This list could go on ad infinitum. Start a list of your own and note the many indications that let you know that your health has improved.

NOTABLE CONCERNS

Once you begin to practice God's Health Laws, your overall health and strength will be greatly improved. But, your body will <u>not</u> become infallible. You still may experience health problems but they will be a lot less dramatic than noted in people who do not follow the health laws.

One major concern is that other people will observe you very closely, they may actually mock or taunt you anytime they detect the slightest problem with your health. Some people will seize every opportunity to discredit you or the effectiveness of the health laws.

> **EXAMPLE:** If you are heard to say something as simple as, "I am tired", you may be accused of not following the health laws or the statement will be used to discredit the effectiveness of the whole plan. If anything ever happens to anyone else who professes to follow the health laws, it will be brought to your attention. You may be questioned by your acquaintances as if you were on trial. It will not matter that you do not know the person or that you have no idea of the circumstances surrounding their situation.

Do not allow mockers to deter you or interfere with your improved life style. Remember, you don't really have to prove anything to anyone else. You will actually feel much better and you will be able to see great improvements in your health. The chances are that others will also notice improvements. Some will mention it to you and others will not. Do not waste precious time trying to determine why people respond as they do, just continue to follow God's health laws.

SPECIAL NOTE

Leg 16, "Weight Management: A Heavy Problem, A Major Benefit of Following the Health Laws", pages 215-220, deals with overweight. A whole leg is devoted to this problem because of its prevalence in our society. This is by no means an indication that people who are either the correct weight or who are underweight have no need to follow the health laws.

When people who are underweight begin practicing the health laws, they begin to gain weight and eventually reach the size which is correct for their height and bone structure.

People who are already at the correct weight for their height and bone structure will still be able to notice improvements in their health in all other areas mentioned when they follow the health laws.

IN SEARCH *OF*

THE FOUNTAIN OF YOUTH

Section IV.

EVERYDAY PROBLEMS FIND SOLUTIONS THROUGH GOD'S COMMANDMENTS, LAWS, STATUES, AND PRINCIPLES

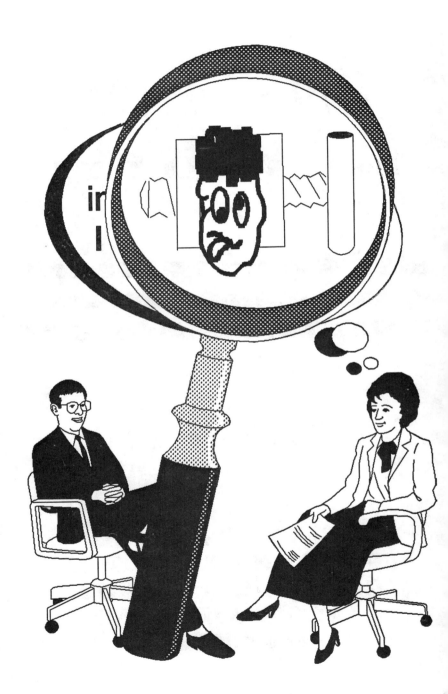

LEG 15

GOD'S HEALTH LAWS: THE PERFECT TOOLS FOR STRESS MANAGEMENT

S INCE people recognize the fact that there is an excess of tension and discomfort within our society, STRESS MANAGEMENT has become an extremely popular subject. For this reason, over the past several years, the author has had the opportunity to deliver many presentations on *STRESS MANAGEMENT* throughout the community. Most presentations are scheduled for about one hour followed by about twenty or thirty minutes of questions and answers. The questions can be answered in the allotted time; but, because the information is very different from what participants are accustomed to hearing, a lot of time is required to <u>explain</u> the answers. In a typical presentation, the limited time has prevented adequate explanations for the answers given.

This can be considered as the written version of a typical **STRESS MANAGEMENT** presentation which includes a basic overview of stress and answers to the most frequently asked questions about stress.

UNDERSTANDING STRESS MANAGEMENT

FAR REACHING CONSEQUENCES

T HE following is a typical beginning for a **STRESS MANAGEMENT** presentation.

Stress Management is both **SIMPLE** and **COMPLEX.** It is **SIMPLE** because the principles are easily understood and accessible to all. It is **COMPLEX** because when followed, the principles have very far-reaching (almost unbelievable) consequences.

As a matter of fact, if today, everyone in the United States decided to manage their **STRESS,** the United States would **NOT** be recognizable a year from now.

Some possible differences would include:

- a state of peace and tranquility instead of restlessness.

- no "processed" food companies.

- no tobacco companies.

- no television commercials containing conflicts between the major fast food chains, as they would all be out of business.

- no fights between the major cola and soft drink companies, as they would also all be out of business.

- no liquor stores.

- no jails.

- very few hospitals.

- longer life expectancy (even today the average person could live about 120 years).

WHAT IS STRESS?

After getting the audience's attention with some of the preceding statements, the questions are asked, "When you hear the word **STRESS** what does it mean to you? What kinds of things do you think about?"

People give several typical answers which can be categorized as stressful situations or physical symptoms.

I.   STRESSFUL SITUATIONS:

- new assignments at work or school.

- preparing for a report or presentation.

- working when you are short of staff.

- problems with employees.

- problems with the boss.

- having to work late when you have made other plans.

- being late for work or school.

- driving in bumper-to-bumper traffic.

- having to deal with disobedient children.

- difficulties with parents.

- having to deal with problems which seem to have no end and no answers.

- family problems.

- having more things to do than you can possibly get done within the allotted time.

- problems with in-laws.

II   **PHYSICAL SYMPTOMS:**

- nervousness.

- headaches.

- ulcers.

- irritability.

- nervous stomach.

- chest pains.

Interestingly, all comments are correct because all of the situations and symptoms are related to stress, even though they are not actually stress itself.

Stress is the _**RESPONSE**_ that the body makes to any internal or external change that it is able to detect. When any of the situations listed in the first group of typical answers occurs, the body will respond; the **RESPONSE** that the body makes to the situations is **STRESS.**   For this reason, the situations listed are stressors. A stressor is the

the actual event or stimuli which occurs and causes the body to respond.

In the second set of typical answers, you will find some of the end results of the body being, **too frequently**, put in a position to have to respond to stressful events without sufficient relief.

HOW DOES THE BODY RESPOND TO STRESS?

Physiologically the body responds to stress by way of the autonomic nervous system. The autonomic nervous system is **"functionally"** divided into two sections which work antagonistically to each other--the sympathetic and the parasympathetic nervous systems. They work like a seesaw. When the sympathetic nervous system is activated the parasympathetic nervous system is inactive and vice-versa.

Activation of the sympathetic nervous system means all of the systems of the body are affected and they respond as follows:

CIRCULATORY SYSTEM - The blood pressure, pulse, and heart rate all go up.

RESPIRATORY SYSTEM - The rate of breathing is increased.

NERVOUS SYSTEM - The senses become impaired, there is a jittery feeling accompanied by irritability.

MUSCULAR SYSTEM - The body is prepared for movement. The skeletal muscles become tense and the smooth muscles relax.

DIGESTIVE SYSTEM - The stomach has the feeling of being all tied up in knots.

ENDOCRINE SYSTEM - The glands dump hormones (such as adrenalin, the fight or flight hormone) into the blood stream at an accelerated rate. The pancreas also dumps increased doses of insulin.

URINARY SYSTEM - The smooth muscles begin to relax. The muscles which control the sphincters of the bladder and the ureters are smooth muscles; therefore, they relax, creating the need to urinate more frequently.

REPRODUCTIVE SYSTEM - Normal functioning is impaired by stress.

SKELETAL SYSTEM - Blood cells are actually made in the marrow of certain bones. Normal functioning of this system is impaired by stress.

All of the above changes occur as a result of activating the sympathetic part of the autonomic nervous system. The brain notes when the vital signs are too high or too low. When it detects an abnormality, it sends signals to activate the proper processes to counteract the abnormality. **THE BODY BEGINS TO RETURN TO NORMAL THROUGH THE ACTIVATION OF THE PARA- SYMPATHETIC NERVOUS SYSTEM.**

Usually, day-by-day, the response to stress is very subtle. The body actually responds to the fact that something has changed, rather than to the event itself.

Basically, most parts of the system are unable to differentiate between that which is considered good and that which is considered bad. Therefore, when bad things happen to us we respond; and, when good things happen to us we respond the same way. The body simply responds to change.

STAGES OF STRESS

Our bodies are naturally designed to respond to stimuli (stressful events). Therefore, in all responses we have the following stages occurring.

- **PERCEPTION** - (conscious or subconscious) the stage in which the body and/or mind moves to a state of awareness that some event has occurred or is about to occur.

- **ONSET** - activation of the sympathetic nervous system.

- **STIMULATION OF THE VARIOUS BODY SYSTEMS** - all of the systems of the body are stimulated to a very high level of activity. If this stage is prolonged, organ damage can result.

- *RECOVERY* - the process by which the parasympathetic nervous system works to slow the activities in the systems of the body. This causes the body functions to return to the state that existed prior to the perception of the stimuli.

TWO BROAD CATEGORIES OF STRESS

- *REGULAR* - every event perceived by the body elicits a stress response. Regular stress is a normal series of responses. Recovery always occurs after each response.

- *CHRONIC* - a continuous series of responses in which recovery is not complete. The system does not return to normal after each stressful episode.

BASIC FACTS ABOUT STRESS

There are certain facts about **STRESS** that are important to our understanding of the **Stress** process.

- Stress is a <u>**NORMAL**</u> part of human existence. God created the body to respond to stimuli. Responding to stimuli through the nervous system is how we experience love, hate, fear, joy, pain, sorrow, and happiness.

■ Prolonged stress **LOWERS THE BODY'S RESISTANCE TO DISEASES**. The body fights disease by the proper functioning of the various systems. Prolonged stress interferes with proper functioning of the systems.

■ The brain **(MIND) IS FULLY CAPABLE OF ACTIVATING A FULL STRESS RESPONSE**. This can happen even though the stimulating event may be long past or totally unreal. This means that we can remember a past event or anticipate an event, activate the sympathetic nervous system; and thus, become very stressed.

■ Even though the amount of stress in one's life can be managed and regulated, **IT IS NOT POSSIBLE FOR US TO ELIMINATE ALL STRESS**. The elimination of all stress means that the body would respond to nothing. No response at all occurs only in death.

■ The body is **DESIGNED TO DEAL WITH SOME STRESS, EVEN A LOT OF STRESS**, but there can be too much stress. We human beings have something built into our systems similar to a "stress threshold". Once the level of stress moves above the stress threshold, serious problems can occur.

Let us imagine that the human stress threshold can expand from 1 (no resistance from the negative effects of stress) to 100 (the maximum resistance to stress). Let us further imagine that most people have a stress threshold between 60 - 80; some may be able to withstand the negative effects of stress by having a threshold as high as 100 and still others may be able to tolerate very little stress because their threshold is far below 60.

Each stressful event registers a certain number of points or carries a certain amount of weight on our stress scales. The weight of any particular event will vary depending on the event itself, extenuating circumstances surrounding the event, and the personality of the person experiencing the situation.

Two people can experience the same stressful event. It is possible for one to be almost totally wiped out and the other to be almost unaffected.

Stress is additive. It builds or rises to a certain level in the body if it is not relieved. Over a period of time we can only take a certain amount of unrelieved stress. Then, something has to give.

When stress builds to the threshold level, the individual will experience a "stress overflow" which expresses itself in the form of physical, mental, or spiritual problems.

When we receive relief from a stressful event, it is eliminated and **will not** have a cumulative negative effect against the system.

When stress is unrelieved, it builds and **does** have a cumulative, negative effect upon the system.

Too much stress can create numerous problems. It can cripple or even kill. Excessive stress (stress which is high but does not go beyond the threshold) can become a chronic situation.

LIFE'S CIRCLE OF CONTROL

If we were to draw a pie chart and try to include all of the things which influence our health, age at death, and fate in other areas; it would look something like the chart in figure 1 on page 201. This chart is an estimate and is not designed from scientific measurement.

Of course, we readily acknowledge that our God has total control. We know that the wind can't blow nor a leaf fall to the ground until He gives His divine **"OKAY"**. But He does delegate to us a certain amount of control and responsibility over our own health and well-being. He has not given us complete control over everything but we do have complete control over whether or not we choose to live within the design that He has given our systems.

The things in this life which influence health, but which are not under our control, are: sex, age, heredity, health care systems, environment, and culture and background. Our lifestyles are basically under our own control.

CIRCLE OF CONTROL EXPLORED

■   *Sex* - influences the diseases that we may get in that a woman will never have prostate disease and a man will never be bothered with ovarian cancer.

Life's Circle of Control

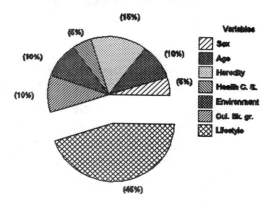

Figure 1

■ *Age* - influences our health in that the body seems to have a built-in time clock inside the cells. Even if disease does not come, under normal circumstances (in our time period), the human body will usually not live past 70 to 90 years. Scientists have said that even under the most ideal circumstances the body will not live beyond 120 or 130 years (see Genesis 6:3). Some have quoted the life span to be as long as 150. This is not very long at all when one considers the fact that God's original plan was for us to live forever.

- *Heredity* - deals with the genes that we all receive from our parents at conception. Genes can carry weaknesses for certain diseases. Such conditions as heart disease, diabetes, and cancer are known to "run in families".

- *Health Care Systems* - have a different kind of influence over our health. The community teaching programs or warnings set forth by various organizations can have a definite influence upon our health. They also have a big part to play once a condition has been diagnosed. Helpful information, excellent health care, and sound medical advice all have a tremendously positive effect on our fate and can actually reverse serious diseases. Of course, there are also the nosocomial diseases, medical misjudgments, or sincere errors which can lead to tragic results.

- *Environment* - influences health dramatically. It is a known fact that (all other things being equal) someone who lives in a "country" area breathing fresh, clean, clear air will live longer than a city dweller who lives next door to a chemical plant.

- *Culture and background* - deals with social and economic statuses and geographical locations. An individual living in a "third world" country where sanitation is poor and medical intervention is almost unheard of, is at a greater risk of developing a serious illness at a very early age and dying prematurely than a person living in a more developed country.

Also, because of stereotyping and discrimination, minorities typically experience far more stress than others in society.

■ *Lifestyle* -   is the one element which has the greatest influence over our health, the type diseases we get, the severity of the diseases, how soon we will get the diseases and whether or not we will succumb to the disease, age of death, and fate in other areas.

 LIFESTYLE   refers to the list of activities which one performs from moment-to-moment, hour-to-hour, day-to-day, and on-and-on. Let us list the things that we do from day-to-day and moment-to-moment, etc. We eat, sleep, drink, think, breath, move muscles, work, make decisions and develop attitudes; the exact activities listed in the health laws.

Two major points about lifestyle are:

■   Our lifestyles have a greater influence over our fate than any other variables mentioned thus far.

■   We have more control over our lifestyles than any of the variables mentioned thus far.

BASIC CAUSES OF STRESS

Stress is the response that the body makes to changes. The events which cause the body to respond are stressors. If we look at all of the events which cause us to respond and group them, we would come up with the categories that follow:

■   *CONFLICT* - a situation arises in which one must choose between two or more things. These things may be equally desirable or equally undesirable, but which ever one is chosen, the others are automatically eliminated as possible choices.

 <u>EXAMPLE</u>: Consider the employee who works on a job where overtime is available periodically. This person is willing to work long hours or come in on scheduled off days. He has informed all supervisors of this and has asked to be placed on a call list. He is planning to use the extra money, earned from working overtime, for a special trip. He counts each hour of overtime as one step closer to his goal.

 Several weeks have elapsed and no overtime has been available. He left work Wednesday afternoon scheduled for two special days off plus his two regular off days. He offered to work Thursday and Friday and take the pay rather than the time. He was told that this was unnecessary.

 Wednesday evening, upon leaving work, he runs several errands which were long overdue. Later, he and some friends go bowling and wind up staying much longer than usual. Finally, he arrives home and being unable to sleep, stays up and watches the late movie. Around 3:00 A. M., he falls asleep.

Wouldn't you know it, the phone rings at 6:00 a.m. It is one of his supervisors. Some of the machinery broke down during the night and they will be short of help after all. He is needed to come in right away. "Not only will you be able to put in the extra eight hours, but it will be very late when you get off tonight."

This is a situation in which options are equally desirable and equally undesirable at the same time.

OPTION 1. Get up and go to work.
Desirable: He would earn the extra money needed, help out on the job and win favor with the supervisors.
Undesirable: He is too physically tired to get up and go to work. He may fall asleep on the job or make some gross error and lose favor with the supervisors or even put his job in jeopardy.

OPTION 2: Stay home.

> **Desirable:** He will be able to obtain the sleep that he needs so much.
>
> **Undesirable:** He will miss out on the extra money, lose the opportunity to help out on the job, lose favor with the supervisors, and possibly lose future opportunities to earn overtime.

This is a conflicting situation. Which choice should he make?

■   *FRUSTRATION* - occurs when a decision has been made to follow a specific plan or to do a certain job. One, several, or all of the steps in the plan have been blocked, causing the whole plan or job to be thwarted or ineffective.

> <u>EXAMPLE:</u> A certain employee has been late six times in the last four weeks. She has received a warning from her supervisor, "One more incidence of tardiness and disciplinary action will be taken." The employee thinks it over and decides that the supervisor really is right and she has been wrong. So, in order to correct her behavior, she will make sure that she is on time for work from now on.
>
> She thinks through her daily routine, and makes a list of all of the things that she could do at night instead of in the morning

on her way to work. This should save a lot of time each morning. Her list states that she will make sure that her clothes and shoes are ready. She will always get gas the evenings before instead of the next morning. She will make sure that she goes to bed at a certain time each night, and she will set her alarm clock for one hour earlier.

She did all of these things and the next morning the alarm clock went off as planned--an hour earlier. But, her body was just not accustomed to getting up at that time. So, she decided to just rest for a few more moments. She intended to hit the snooze button, but accidently turned off the whole alarm system. Finally, she wakes up thinking that she has gotten only a few minutes of extra sleep when; actually, she has received more than an hour of additional sleep.

When she discovers that she has overslept, she makes a mad dash for the bathroom and gets her shower and gets dressed. "Well", she thinks, "It really does help that I have done all of those other things. I may be on time after all."

She jumps in her car and heads for the expressway. Wouldn't you know it, a wreck or something has occurred. There is a very long line of cars waiting on the ramp to get on the expressway. There is no way that she can make it if she tries to go this route. She remembers an alternate route and finally arrives at work a few minutes before time to hit the time clock. Is it possible that she can still make it? She rushes inside the building and steps up to the elevator. Just as she pushes the button, she notices the "out-of-order" sign pasted to the door. She arrives at her work station a few minutes late.

This employee set the goal that she would be on time for work. She made plans to accomplish this goal, but several steps in the plan were blocked; thus, destroying the whole plan.

This person is frustrated.

■   ***PRESSURE*** - deals with a condition in which there is too much of a demand on the available resources, and the demands are all coming at the same time. Resources can be defined as time, energy, money, and intellect.

> **EXAMPLE:** A young working mother of three small children decided to return to school to increase job opportunities. One afternoon, she realizes that she has to prepare dinner for the family, study for an exam scheduled for

the next day, work on a project that she brought home from her job (this project must be turned in the first thing the next morning), and iron her clothes and the children's clothes for the next day.

She just received a call from her in-laws. They are visiting a friend in the neighborhood and would like to drop in for a few moments to visit with the kids.

Her husband has not arrived home since he had to work late.

The house is a mess.

This young mother is under pressure. Everything and everybody seem to be demanding her time, energy, and attention all at the same time.

■ *SURPRISE* - a sudden emotional shock or to suddenly become aware of the unexpected.

EXAMPLE: A young married couple has decided that they will limit their family to their one child. They are practicing birth control. The wife feels ill, goes to her physician for a check-up, and learns that she is pregnant.

SURPRISE ! !.

■   *CONSTANT ANXIETY* - dreadful, sometimes chronic, anticipation of the worse--a constant state of fearfulness.

> **EXAMPLE:** A middle aged woman describes herself as being a "nervous wreck". She is easily excited and always feels that the very "worst" is going to happen. She returns home after a shopping trip and finds a message on her answering machine from her youngest son. He is attending college in another state. His message was, "Hi mom, call me as soon as you get home, I have some exciting news for you."
>
> She immediately becomes jittery and nervous. She has to call a neighbor over to stay with her while she returns her son's call. When she finally gets up the nerves to return his call, she learns that he has gotten a summer job and will not be coming home as usual.
>
> After the call, she begins thinking of all of the really "terrible" things that could happen to him if he does not come home as usual. She becomes so agitated that she decides to go to her physician for a check-up. Her blood pressure and pulse are elevated. She then begins to worry about her health.

This woman is constantly anxious. In all events she assumes that the worst will occur.

■   ***EXTREME PLEASURE*** - the really pleasurable and exciting things that happen to us from time to time.

> **EXAMPLE**: A man wins the lottery for one million dollars. Upon receiving the news, he becomes so excited that he suffers a heart attack and must be rushed to the closest emergency room.

This experience was extreme pleasure but too stressful for his system.

■   ***INTENSE PERSONALITY TYPES*** - an extremely intense response to situations. Some people, for whatever reason, respond to stressful events more dramatically than others.

> **EXAMPLE**: The police radar is hidden on a busy street.   Many cars are stopped for exceeding the speed limit. Most of the people ticketed become upset at first, but soon acknowledge that they were, in fact, speeding. They take their tickets and go on their way.
>
> One man who also received a ticket for exceeding the speed limit argued that he was totally innocent as long as it was tolerated by the officer. He felt that the ticket was unjustified.

He sulked and stayed angry about the incident for several weeks. He told the story over and over to friends and co-workers and insisted that he was the victim of a gross miscarriage of justice.

He responded more intensely to the situation than normal.

All of the above situations caused stress. But stress must be **MANAGED** because it can not be totally eliminated.

MANAGING STRESS-VERSUS-ELIMINATING IT

Absolutely **NO** stress means that the system makes **NO** response to anything (this is death).

For simplification, we will divide the stressors into two major classifications:

(1.) THE UNAVOIDABLE STRESSORS - those events which occur regardless of our attempts to avoid them. We are unable to prevent them or to control them.

(2.) THE UNNECESSARY STRESSORS - stressful events which occur that could have been prevented.

Our objective is to eliminate all of the unnecessary stressors, by following God's health laws, in order to make the body strong enough to deal with the unavoidable stressors.

STRESS SUMMARY

The main thing that we need to remember about stress is that it is normal. All instances of change cause a central nervous system reaction. The body is designed to respond a certain way when change occurs.

There are many events which can occur over which we have no control. Also, it is noted that there are too many events which occur over which we do not want control.

Even if we really wanted to eliminate all of the things that we consider bad, we could not. There is no way that we can remove all stress from our lives. To remove all of the stress from our lives is for us to die.

In any case, we get into trouble when stressful events occur too often. They take a toll on our bodies and "wear us out".

Anyone who develops the attitude that he or she will live within the body's design by incorporating the health laws into his or her lifestyle, will experience the benefits listed at the end of Leg 15, "What Can We Expect From Following The Health Laws?" (see page 179-185). Living outside of the body's design creates undue stress on all organs and systems of the body. When we disregard the health laws for a long period of time our perception of life and all circumstances becomes severely altered.

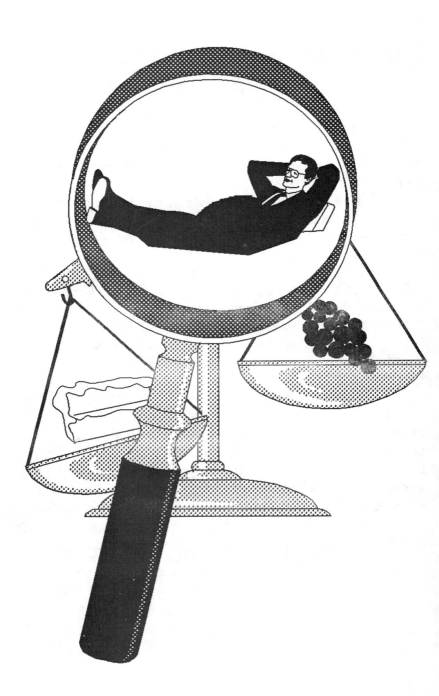

LEG 16

WEIGHT MANAGEMENT: A HEAVY PROBLEM

A MAJOR BENEFIT OF FOLLOWING THE HEALTH LAWS

O F the approximately 250 million people in America, more than 80 million are overweight. Being over-weight means carrying around more pounds than the frame and internal organs can support. Every book on weight management recommends a reduction in the amount of food taken in and an increase in the amount of

215

energy expended. People who are knowledgeable about health recommend "A CHANGE IN LIFESTYLE" rather than a "REDUCTION DIET" for a specified period of time. Adopting the HEALTH LAWS outlined in Leg 13 of this book is the very best Lifestyle change available. Once these principles are practiced for a while, the body will automatically move to its proper weight.

Weight Management is special because it comes with the precautions or concerns outlined below.

PHYSICAL CONCERNS ASSOCIATED WITH WEIGHT LOSS

■ The direction of weight loss is usually downward. Your figure will probably be disproportionate during the weight loss process. Your upper extremities, for a while, may be somewhat smaller than the lower extremities.

■ Weight loss is somewhat slow, but permanent if the health laws are followed permanently.

■ Typically, overweight people have an excess of water as well as fat. You will lose the excess water prior to or along with the fat in the early stages of the process. During this period, the rate of weight loss may be very rapid. Once the excess fluid is gone, the rate of weight loss will begin to slow down.

■ Practicing the health laws will cause you to develop muscle tissue as you lose the fatty tissue and water. Since muscle tissue weighs more than fatty tissue and water, but is much less bulky than fat tissue, it is possible for you to be much slimmer; yet, weigh more than you did when you were fatter. In other words, you will be slimmer but the scales won't show it at all times.

■ Typically, women will **NOT** lose weight just prior to their monthly cycle. It is possible for one to follow all of the health laws and actually gain weight at this particular time. Don't despair, the extra weight is just the body holding water. Continue with your lifestyle plan and the water weight will leave. A woman who follows all of the health laws will not gain as much water weight during this time as one who does not. In either case, the excess water will leave either during or after the monthly cycle.

■ There is one concern that many people have when they begin to lose weight--loose sagging skin (especially in the abdominal area and on the upper arms). Following all of the health laws also reduces this problem. Sagging flesh in the abdominal area will be greatly reduced by the following practices: never filling the stomach beyond its capacity, gently holding the stomach muscles in at all times, not taking water or other liquids with meals, and performing the exercises for the abdominal muscles listed on page 154 & 155.

PSYCHOLOGICAL CONCERNS OF WEIGHT LOSS

- You must make a "total" commitment to take control of your own lifestyle.

- The best possible method of weight management does not include a "diet" which you will be on for a while; then, go back to old habits and find all of the lost pounds. With the plan to follow the health laws, you make a total change from unhealthy habits to healthy ones.

- You must accept the fact that weight loss is a slow process.

- Remember, everyone will not automatically think that you look better thin. Family, friends, neighbors, co-workers, and other associates may think that you looked much better before you lost weight than you do at your new size. They will make statements such as, "You look **FUNNY** now that you are smaller. I liked you better fat. Your face was so pretty before; now, its much too narrow.

You look sick, maybe you are losing too fast. I don't see where you have lost any at all." They will tempt you with food that does not fit into your plan and insist that, "this little piece won't hurt you." The motivation for such behavior may be a sincere concern, jealousy, or curiosity. Some people think that thin is prettier, others really think that fat is prettier. Beauty is in the eyes of the beholder. We all know that being the correct weight is healthier than being overweight. Don't waste your precious time trying to figure out their motivation, just **"STICK TO YOUR PLAN."**

■ Lose weight for yourself, your own health, appearance, etc. In other words, **"DO IT FOR YOU."** Never lose weight to please any one else, or to get anyone's attention.

■ Prepare for special occasions. All special occasions focus on food: holidays, birthdays, homecomings, weddings, family reunions, parties, and even funerals. Practice the survival techniques such as: eating only the foods that fit into your food plan and eating only at the times specified in your plan. Compliment the Hostess on the items that you can eat. If someone insists that you "simply must taste this", stand your ground. If it does not fit into your food plan, continue to refuse. If it does fit into your food plan; but, the time is wrong, consider taking it with you on the "freeze now, eat later" plan. Never,

Never, Never omit meals because you are invited to some function later in the evening.

■ If your new lifestyle and lowered weight makes it necessary for you to be "different" from most people, accept the fact that you are different. Consider yourself to be in good company. All of God's people are "supposed" to be different--even **peculiar"**.

> "And the LORD hath avouched thee this day to be his peculiar people, as he hath promised thee, and that thou shouldest keep all his commandments;"
> Deuteronomy 26:18

■ Understand that once you are a thin person your problems will not suddenly begin to solve themselves. Weight management is just one of the bonuses of following all of the Health Laws. It is not a "cure-all" for all of life's problems.

Now that you have the facts, proceed with a plan to practice the health laws. This will lead to a slimmer, healthier you.

LEG 17

WHAT'S THE TROUBLE WITH KIDS TODAY?

Picture this:

SCENE ONE

There is this loud music playing. Three or four teenagers are sitting around the room in some awkward positions. One or two others are making some stupid movements to the music. They are all wearing some very funny-looking clothes. Each is dressed in an outfit that is big enough for at least

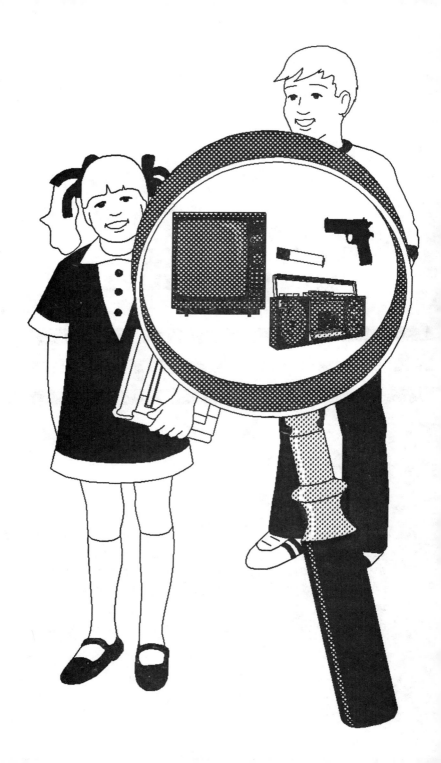

one other person to get into it with him. The room is in total disarray. Popcorn, pillows, and other unsightly things are all over the sofa and floor.

SCENE TWO

In walks dad. On his face you read the signs of total disbelief. He attempts to speak to one of the teenagers who is oblivious to his presence. Finally, he walks into another room and the theme song for the program begins to play, "What's The Trouble With Kids Today?"

It has been so long ago that my memory of the situation is not so clear; but, this scene surely is very similar to one of the television shows that I watched several years back. Though I can't remember much of the program, the words in the theme song have stuck in my memory. Since that time, whenever I hear or read something about the things that teenagers are doing and the trouble they are getting into (teenage pregnancies, violent crimes, drugs, suicide) the words in that song come back to my mind and I think, "LORD, WHAT'S THE TROUBLE WITH KIDS TODAY?"

I can also remember reading an article in the magazine of the local Sunday newspaper. It was several years ago, but I do remember some of the information that was presented. It seemed to be a comparative analysis of what was happening with teenagers at the time of the article and what was happening to them twenty years earlier.

It was pointed out that twenty years before the article, the biggest problems that teachers had with students were: coming to class late, hitting or pushing each other in the cafeteria line, not finishing homework, and fistfights on the playground.

At the time of the article teachers cited their major problems with kids as: students carrying weapons such as switchblades and hand guns, teen pregnancies, illegal drugs being sold and used in the schools, students engaging in sexual activities on school premises, and physical attacks on teachers as well as students.

I have heard some teachers say that students arrive for classes so "stoned" (high on drugs) that the teachers wonder how they made it there. As I ponder over this information, once again the words in that song come back to me and I wonder, "LORD, WHAT'S THE TROUBLE WITH KIDS TODAY?"

I remember hearing a sermon in which the theme was, "Earth Has No Sorrow That Heaven Cannot Heal". The speaker made the point that there is no problem for which the Bible does not carry an answer. So I turned to the Scriptures to shed some light on these problems with kids that plagued me so much. One scripture that caught my eye was found in Ecclesiastes.

> "The thing that hath been, it is that which shall be; and that which is done is that which shall be done: and there is no new thing under the sun."

Ecclesiastes 1:9

As I looked at what has been happening to our youth for the past few years, and looked at what was happening twenty to twenty-five years ago, I was almost tempted to differ with that scripture. But, of course; as always, a closer observation confirms that the scripture is correct.

A study of Child Development reveals that children mature through a succession of developmental stages with each stage bringing its own problems and stresses and requiring additional capabilities than before.   The succeeding stage takes what was learned from previous experiences and transforms it into information that can be used to solve problems in the present. The child, through a very systematic process, becomes more competent and capable in the various areas of functioning.

It is the job of the parents, teachers, and others in the child's environment to direct, support, teach, and be positive role models for the child as he or she moves through each stage.

As I thought of the kids today, I reflected on my own childhood. I can remember that when I was growing up, raising children did not seem to be a job left solely to parents. Uncles, aunts, grandparents, and well meaning neighbors and friends all had a role to play.

I can remember walking to school when I was in the first grade. Almost every adult person that I passed took an interest in my welfare. If it was cold, they wanted to know where my scarf and gloves were. If it was raining, they questioned me if I didn't have an umbrella. They watched as I crossed the street and cautioned me to look both ways. They made us kids stop fighting on the way home from school.

If we received a spanking at school, we didn't run home to tell mother so that she could file a law suit against the teacher. We didn't tell her at all and prayed that no one else would. We didn't want her to know because she would give us another spanking for behaving in such a manner that made us deserve the first one.

When we arrived home from school, we were greeted by mother or some other adult who had a warm meal prepared. If for some reason no adult was available to greet us, we had to go to a neighbor's house or to the home of a relative or a friend of the family. Yes, twenty or thirty years ago, raising kids was everyone's responsibility. My observation is that this attitude is not so prevalent today.

Today, in most American homes, both parents work. The number of households headed by single parents is steadily growing. Schools are finding that most kids do not get a healthy breakfast in the mornings and are left to feast on "junk food" throughout the day and at night. It is not at all unusual for kids to come home from school to an empty house. This situation is so frequent that such children have been given the name "latch-key kids".

In my experience as a counselor, I have had the opportunity to talk to children individually and in groups. I find that many children do not trust adults. They feel that adults give them inaccurate information when important questions are asked.

Young people are left alone to ponder over such questions as: "Does God really exist? If He does exist, where is He? What happens to people when they die? Why is there pain and suffering? What is the purpose of life and the meaning of human existence?"

While it is totally true that there is "no new thing under the sun", the responses that kids have to make to the environment have dramatically increased. As mentioned throughout this book, all things are chemical and electrical. People have learned to take chemistry and electricity and rearrange it to bring about numerous gadgets and instruments, making the environment appear a lot more complex and confusing. Such gadgets are: automobiles, radios, televisions, VCRs, computers, guns, pills, ad infinitum.

As we look at the total picture:

- confusion related to teleological and eschatological questions,

- a decrease in the amount of direction, support, and environmental structure from adults,

- the peer pressure,

- the lack of trust of adults,

- the dramatic increase in the amount of gadgets in the environment to which kids of today must react;

a lot of light is shed on the question, "What's the trouble with kids today?"

QUESTION: "What's The Trouble With Kids Today?"

ANSWER: They need to possess a feeling of being loved, a knowledge of God's love, loving parents, prayer, guidance, a structured environment, direction, and the knowledge of God's word (including His Health Laws).

As the sermon pointed out, Earth has no sorrow that heaven cannot heal, and the answers to all of life's problems really are found in the Holy Scriptures.

"O God, thou hast taught me from my youth: and hitherto have I declared thy wondrous works."
Psalms 71:17

"Train up a child in the way he should go: and when he is old, he will not depart from it."
Proverbs 22:6

"And all thy children shall be taught of the LORD; and great shall be the peace of thy children."
Isaiah 54:13

IN Sᴇᴀʀᴄʜ *OF*

Tʜᴇ Fᴏᴜɴᴛᴀɪɴ Oꜰ Yᴏᴜᴛʜ

Section V.

THE GREATEST GIFT

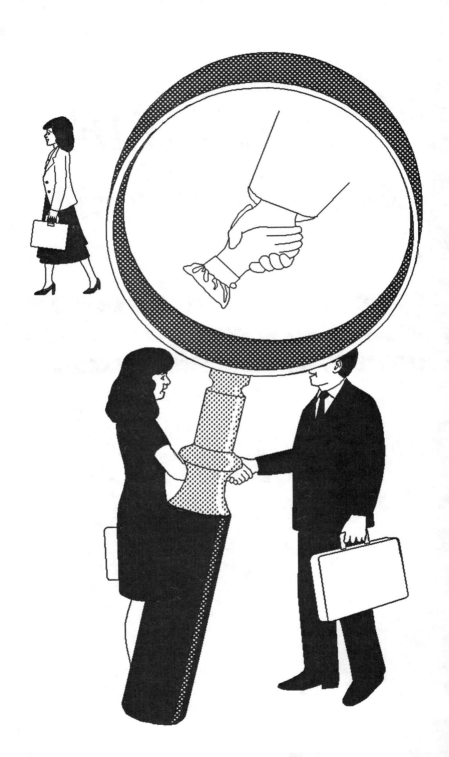

LEG 18

THE ULTIMATE PRINCIPLE OF HEALTH

A PERSONAL RELATIONSHIP WITH GOD: FAITH, TRUST, OBEDIENCE, STUDY, PRAYER, and UNSELFISH SERVICE

W HAT is the greatest gift that a human being can receive? You probably think that the answer that we are looking for is health because that's been the focus of this entire book. We all agree that health is of the utmost importance.

Health actually exists on a continuum. To be healthy the individual must gravitate toward wellness. Wellness is an active state of being. There is nothing passive about it. It is an exuberant burst of energy and activity which makes one **WANT** to live life to the fullest. Ultimate health requires a complete integration and interrelatedness of the mind, body, and spirit. The individual enters a growth process which leads him or her to the highest level of well-being. The activities which render one to be actively involved in wellness all involve practicing the health laws presented in Leg 13 of our journey, pages 119-177.

A serious concern is the fact that regardless of how healthy one is, there will come a time when the precious **FOUNTAIN OF YOUTH** that we have discovered will stop spurting forth its healthful elixir. This means that, at best, no matter how happy or how healthy we are, we are limited to a finite number of years here on planet earth. Even if we do everything discussed thus far; eventually, when the biological clock runs out, we die. No matter how beautifully and perfectly we try to paint the picture of life and good health, we still have the ugly, dreadful finality of death to look forward to.

Well, there may be hope yet. In the Introduction, page xvi, we talked about the possibility of finding a **FOUNTAIN OF YOUTH** that had the capability of allowing us to live forever.

Now we will answer the question asked at the beginning of this Leg of our journey, **"What is the greatest gift that anyone can ever receive?"**

Answer: The **"Greatest Gift" that anyone can ever receive is Jesus Christ** through whom we receive the gift of **"Eternal Life"**.

> "For God so loved the world, that he gave his only begotten Son, that whosoever believeth in him should not perish, but have everlasting life."
> John 3:16

> "Whosoever committeth sin transgresseth also the law: for sin is the transgression of the law."
> I John 3:4

> "For the wages of sin is death; but the gift of God is eternal life through Jesus Christ our Lord."
> Romans 6:23

In Leg 12, page 108, we learned that the major component of God's character is love. The **"Greatest Love" is manifested through The Love** that Jesus expressed for us when He died for us on the cross.

God created us and He **LOVES** us regardless of what we do. But, **HIS ETERNAL LIFE** is **NOT** given to us regardless of what we do. We can have **ETERNAL LIFE** only if we decide to do His will and accept this precious gift that He has offered us by keeping all of His commandments.

"If you love me, keep my commandments."
John 14:15

In order to fulfill the final requirement of the **Fountain of Youth**, we need to look at one more **HEALTH LAW**, the most important one; a personal relationship with God. This is the only way that we will be able to live forever. A personal relationship with God involves Faith, Trust, Obedience, Study, Prayer, and Unselfish Service. Each component of this relationship is of utmost importance.

11. LAW: A PERSONAL RELATIONSHIP
WITH GOD

God created the universe. He is the "LIFE GIVER". There is no existence outside the jurisdiction of the Lord God Almighty. But, God does not force Himself upon us. He gives us the freedom to choose to serve Him, and in turn choose eternal life. Or, we are free to choose the other path available; the one which leads to death and destruction.

If we choose to serve God, we must allow Him to develop a personal relationship with us and help us to grow spiritually. It is through the spirit that the relationship with God develops. It is important for us to remember that just as physical growth is a step-by-step process, so it is with spiritual growth.

A.   REFERENCE SCRIPTURE(S)

FAITH

"All things were made by him; and without him was not any thing made that was made."
John 1:3

"Now faith is the substance of things hoped for, the evidence of things not seen."
Hebrews 11:1

"NOW THE JUST SHALL LIVE BY FAITH: BUT IF ANY MAN DRAW BACK, MY SOUL SHALL HAVE NO PLEASURE IN HIM."
Hebrews 10:38

"But without faith it is impossible to please him: for he that cometh to God must believe that he is, and that he is a rewarder of them that diligently seek him."
Hebrews 11:6

TRUST

"Trust in the LORD and do good; so shalt thou dwell in the land, and verily thou shalt be fed."
Psalms 37:3

"Trust in the LORD for ever; for in the LORD JEHOVAH is everlasting strength:"
Isaiah 26:4

OBEDIENCE

"And Samuel said, Hath the LORD as great delight in burnt offerings and sacrifices, as in obeying the voice of the LORD? Behold, to obey is better than sacrifice, and to hearken than the fat of rams."
I Samuel 15:22

"Then Peter and the other apostles answered and said, We ought to obey God rather than men."
Acts 5:29

"Casting down imaginations, and every high thing that exalteth itself against the knowledge of God, and bringing into captivity every thought to the obedience of Christ;"
II Corinthians 10:5

STUDY

"Study to shew thyself approved unto God, a workman that needeth not to be ashamed, rightly dividing the word of truth."
II Timothy 2:15

PRAYER

"Pray without ceasing."
I Thessalonians 5:17

"After this manner therefore pray ye: Our Father which art in heaven, Hallowed be thy name.
Thy kingdom come. Thy will be done in earth, as it is in heaven.

Give us this day our daily bread.
And forgive us our debts, as we
forgive our debtors.
And lead us not into
temptation, but deliver us from
evil: For thine is the kingdom,
and the power and the glory,
for ever. Amen."
Matthew 6:9-13

UNSELFISH SERVICE

"Pure religion and undefiled
before God is this, To visit the
fatherless and widows in their
affliction, and to keep himself
unspotted before the world."
James 1:27

B.   RATIONALE

As our personal relationship with God develops, we
grow in:

FAITH - the belief that God will do what He says
and that He will do it when He knows it is the best
time to do it. This is an intangible element but we
will be aware of it as it develops.

TRUST - the ability to wait patiently for God to do that which He has promised. Trust is also intangible and will develop with time and experience.

OBEDIENCE - the process of following all of God's commandments, statues, and directions, even when we don't understand why it is necessary for us to do so.

STUDY - reading God's Holy word; thus, allowing Him to communicate with us by providing special instructions and information. It is God's way of talking to us. He teaches us about Himself and gives examples for us to follow as we make decisions day-by-day. Certain Biblical reference books and commentaries should be included in the study periods. It must be remembered that study is of little value without **Faith, Trust, Obedience, and Prayer.**

PRAYER - vertical communication with our God, Lord, Savior, and Creator of the heaven and the earth. It is the breath of the soul. During prayer we talk to God as a friend. The **"ART OF PRAYER"** is developed by the **HOLY SPIRIT.** When prayers are answered, God's promises are reclaimed. Before we pray, He already knows what we **want,** and more importantly, He knows what we **NEED.** Sometimes, what we want is in direct conflict with what we need. He wants to give us the things that are best for us and He knows the best times and circumstances under which to give His gifts. This does not mean that we cannot ask for what we want. It means that God loves us so much that in His divine wisdom, He may not always give us exactly what we ask for.

PRAYER is designed for us to communicate with God and for Him to work out His divine plan in our lives in such a way that we may be able to comprehend His great love and concern for us.

UNSELFISH SERVICE - the process of sharing all resources as directed by the Holy Spirit. Recently, when the last census was taken, a major concern about accuracy was discussed. Census takers knew that the final "head count" would be inaccurate because it is extremely difficult to keep an accurate record of the number of homeless people living in this country. The number of homeless, needy, and hungry people has risen all over the world. If we are to have a personal relationship with Jesus, we must share His concern about these people and minister to them.

So, how concerned is Jesus about the hungry, prisoners, orphans, homeless people, and others who have great needs? We can say with certainty that Jesus feels every hunger pang that a hungry person feels. He cries with every parent who sheds a tear for their children when some of the most simple things cannot be provided. We can say this with absolute certainty because of two facts.

FACT # 1.   When Jesus walked this earth in human form, He actually spent most of His time with those in need. Oh, we know that His main objectives were to demonstrate the great love of the Father, and show us that we can live a sinless life on planet earth. But He accomplished this goal by serving those in need and being homeless himself (Matthew 8:20).

FACT # 2.   Jesus wants to point out the plight of those in need so much that He actually tied salvation (the gift of eternal life) to how each individual treats those in need.

"When the Son of man shall come in his glory, and all the holy angels with him, then shall he sit upon the throne of his glory:
And before him shall be gathered all nations: and he shall separate them one from another, as a shepherd divideth his sheep from the goats:
And he shall set the sheep on his right hand, but the goats on the left.
Then shall the King say unto them on his right, Come, ye blessed of my Father, inherit the kingdom prepared for you from the

foundation of the world: For I was an hungered, and ye gave me meat: I was thirsty, and ye gave me drink: I was a stranger, and ye took me in:

Naked, and ye clothed me: I was sick, and ye visited me: I was in prison, and ye came unto me.

Then shall the righteous answer him saying, LORD, when saw we thee an hungred, and fed thee? or thirsty, and gave thee drink?

When saw we thee a stranger, and took thee in? or naked, and clothed thee?

Or when saw thee sick, or in prison and came unto thee?

And the King shall answer and say unto them, Verily I say unto you, Inasmuch as you have done it unto the least of these my brethren, ye have done it unto me.

Then shall he say unto them on the left hand, Depart from me ye cursed, into everlasting fire, prepared for the devil and his angels:

For I was an hungred, and ye gave me no meat: I was thirsty, and ye gave me no drink: I was a stranger, and ye took me not in: naked, and ye clothed me not: sick and in prison, and ye visited me not.

Then shall they also answer him, saying, LORD, when saw we thee an hungred, or athirst, or a stranger, or naked, or sick, or in prison, and did not minister unto thee?

Then shall he answer them, saying, Verily I say unto you, Inasmuch as ye did it not to one of the least of these, ye did it not to me. And these shall go away into everlasting punishment: but the righteous into life eternal."
Matthew 25 31-46

C.   SUGGESTED METHOD(S) OF PRACTICE

I.   FAITH

Faith is practiced by becoming patient and learning to believe that God will do what He says. It will develop as we pray, study, and obey.

II.   TRUST

Trust is developed by "putting God to the test". We must follow His commandments, even when it is very difficult. We must watch and wait as He takes control. Trust, just as faith, is intangible. It will develop as we pray, study, and obey.

III.   OBEDIENCE

We must make a conscious effort to obey God and keep all of His commandments and statues. As we do this, we will note gradual improvements in our health. If we want to measure the improvements, we can:

■ perform an initial assessment of our present health status (see Appendix).

■ set target goals.

■ keep records of our progress.

■ consciously arrange our circumstances so that we will be able to meet our goals.

EXAMPLE 1 If you plan to walk every day but get off from work too late almost every day, carry a pair of walking shoes to work and keep them there. Select periods of time to walk (breaks and lunchtime, etc.)

EXAMPLE 2 If you have decided to become a vegetarian but are unable to find enough food in the work site cafeteria to maintain a healthy diet, bring your lunch from home.

Continue to monitor your progress. If you fall short of your goals, thank God for what He has already done and ask Him to give you the strength and courage that you need to continue. If you are meeting your goals, thank God for everything that He has done. Ask Him for the strength to continue in His grace.

IV.   STUDY

Set aside specific periods of time when you will be able to concentrate and study **GOD'S WORD** daily and be willing to do what it says in order to:

■   determine where you are in your relationship with God.

■   understand His promises concerning answering prayer.

■   receive an understanding as to how God answers prayer.

Whether you study alone or with a group, always open and end the study session with prayer.

"These were more noble than those in Thessalonica, in that they received the word with all readiness of mind, and searched the scriptures daily, whether those things were so."
Acts 17:11

V.   PRAYER

Our relationship with God is the most important relationship that we will ever have the opportunity to experience. But, as with any other relationship, the key to maintaining the relationship in a positive mode is keeping the lines of communication open.

One of God's avenues for communicating with us is through the Holy Scriptures. The scriptures tell us that: it is God's will that none should perish and that we will all have eternal life, God will not force us into a relationship with Him against our will, and that God never changes.

It is through prayer that God allows us to communicate with Him. Since God won't force the relationship, our prayers assume a very important role in this relationship. For this reason, the scriptures have given us a lot of information concerning all aspects of prayer. Much of this information is presented on the next few pages.

METHODS OF PRAYER

Ask in the name of JESUS.

"And whatsoever ye shall ask in my name, that will I do, that the Father may be glorified in the Son. If ye shall ask any thing in my name, I will do it."
John 14:13-14

Abide by **JESUS'** rules! Keep His commandments and do that which is pleasing in His sight.

"If ye love me, keep my commandments,"
John 14:15

"And whatsoever we ask, we receive of him, because we keep His commandments, and do those things that are pleasing in his sight."
I John 3:22

Ask inside the **"WILL OF GOD"**, believe that your prayers will be answered.

"And all things, whatsoever ye shall ask in prayer, believing, ye shall receive."
Matthew 21:22

We must **BELIEVE** on the **NAME** of **JESUS** and **LOVE** one another.

"And this is his commandment, That we should believe on the name of His Son Jesus Christ,

and love one another, as he
gave us commandment."
I John 3:23

We must belong to our LORD JESUS. We
must abide in Him as He abides in us.

"If ye abide in me, and my
words abide in you, ye shall
ask what ye will, and it shall
be done unto you."
John 15:7

Abide in THE HOLY SPIRIT.

"And he that keepeth his
commandments dwelleth in
him and he in him. And
hereby we know that he
abideth in us, by the Spirit
which he hath given us."
I John 3:24

THE NEED FOR PRAYER

Jesus prayed.

"And He went a little farther, and fell on His face, and prayed, saying, O my Father, if it be possible, let this cup pass from me: nevertheless not as I will, but as thou wilt."
Matthew 26:39

It is only through prayer that we will "yield not to temptation".

"Watch and pray, that ye enter not into temptation: the spirit indeed is willing, but the flesh is weak."
Matthew 26:41

It is through prayer that we gain strength.

"And He spake a parable unto them to this end, that men ought always to pray, and not to faint;"
Luke 18:1

It is through prayer that we find our Lord and Savior.

"Then shall ye call upon me,
and ye shall go and pray unto
me, and I will hearken unto
you.
And ye shall seek me, and find
me, when ye shall search for
me with all your heart."
Jeremiah 29:12-13

HINDRANCES TO ANSWERED PRAYER

HOLDING INIQUITY

"If I regard iniquity in my
heart, the LORD will not hear
me:"
Psalms 66:18

MAKING SELFISH REQUESTS OF GOD

"Ye ask, and receive not,
because ye ask amiss, that ye
may consume it upon your
lusts."
James 4:3

AREAS OF PRAYER

PRAISE

"Let them praise the name of the LORD: for His name alone is excellent; His glory is above the earth and heaven."
Psalms 148:13

THANKSGIVING

"And Mattaniah the son of Micha, the son of Zabdi, the son of Asaph, was the principal to begin the thanksgiving in prayer..."
Nehemiah 11:17

"Let us come before His presence with thanksgiving, and make a joyful noise unto Him with psalms."
Psalms 95:2

CONFESSION (Acknowledging Our Sins)

"And Joshua said unto Achan, My son, give, I pray thee, glory to the LORD God of Israel, and make confession unto Him;....."
Joshua 7:19

"He that covereth his sins shall not prosper: but whoso confesseth and forsaketh them shall have mercy."
Proverbs 28:13

INTERCESSION (Prayer for Others)

"I EXHORT therefore, that, first of all, supplications, prayers, intercessions, and giving of thanks, be made for all men;"
I Timothy 2:1

PETITION (Asking for Specific Things)

"For this child I prayed; and the LORD hath given me my petition which I asked of Him."
I Samuel 1:27

"And if we know that He hear us, whatsoever we ask, we know that we have the petitions that we desired of Him."
I John 5:15

A SPECIAL PRAYER REQUEST

A very special prayer was given to the author by the Holy Spirit. In a dream she had been commissioned by God to defend His character at all costs. She accepted the commission. Upon awakening she became very frightened. The fear was not of others, but of herself for she was aware of her many shortcomings. She prayed, "Oh Lord, I am only human. What if I make a mistake or misinterpret parts of the message as I try to explain it. What if I speak to people too strongly and hurt their feelings. I want to do as you ask, but Lord God, I am not worthy and I am not capable." The Holy Spirit directed her to pray this prayer, share it with her family, and for the whole family to incorporate it into their daily prayer lives.

PRAYER

Dear Lord God, Creator of the heaven and earth, please fill us with your Holy Spirit and be with us always.

Totally control our thoughts at all times.
Fill our minds with only that which YOU want us to think.
Let our eyes see only that which YOU want us to see.

Let our ears hear only that which YOU want us to hear.
Let our tongues speak only that which YOU want us to speak.
Let our mouths and stomachs receive only that which YOU approve.
Let our hands do only that which YOU want us to do.
Guide our feet so that we will go only those places that YOU want us to go.

Give us the strength and guidance to follow all of YOUR Commandments, Laws, Statues, and Principles.

This special prayer request we ask in the name of our Precious Lord and Savior, Jesus Christ.

Amen.

Your most humble servants.

Cora, Jim, Cindy, JEHT, Cid

UNSELFISH SERVICE

Share blessings with those who are less fortunate by sharing your resources, (time, money, energy). Ask God to show you the most efficient ways to accomplish this goal.

When God gives you the opportunity, spend some time with the homeless and others who are less fortunate. Talk with them, pray with them and show them that God loves them so much that He sent you to minister unto them.

> "For the poor shall never cease out of the land: therefore I command thee, saying, Thou shalt open thine hand wide unto thy brother, to thy poor and to the needy, in the land."
> Deuteronomy 15:11

D. Notable Results

Accepting Jesus Christ as Lord and Savior means becoming willing to do as He says which means following all of His commandments and health laws.

In addition to all of the notable results attached at the end of each law presented in Leg 13 of our journey, "A Thorough Search of the Biblical Health Laws" (pages 119-177) and Leg 14, "What Can We Expect From Following The Health Laws" (pages 179-185), we will be able to say with full assurance, "Whatever my lot, Thou hast taught me to say, it is well with my soul."

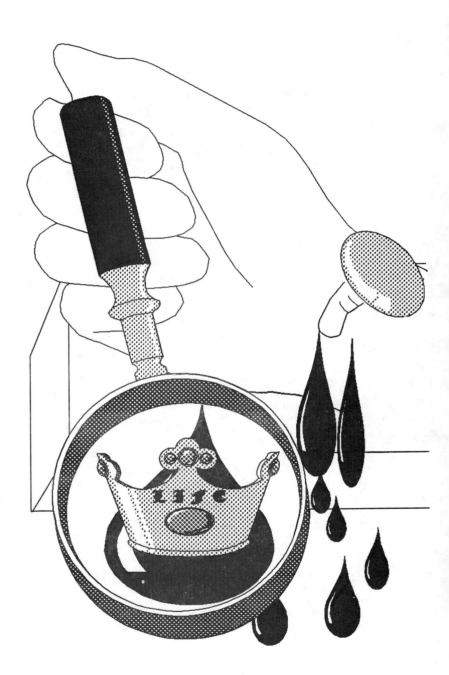

LEG 19

THE ULTIMATE FOUNTAIN OF YOUTH

CLEANSING THROUGH THE
PRECIOUS BLOOD OF JESUS CHRIST:
The Ultimate Fountain of Youth

T rust, Faith, Study, Obedience, Prayer, and Unselfish Service are the six principles that are available to us as the tools with which to build a personal relationship with Christ. Even though the relationship is progressive, Jesus immediately covers us with His blood, the ultimate **FOUNTAIN OF YOUTH.** He washes away our sins and gives us the promise of eternal life.

Eternal life means that **WE WILL NEVER DIE** (John 11:21-26).   Before we become confused with this statement, the fact needs to be brought forth that there are two different types of death. The first death is merely a "sleep" (Matthew 9:18-25) from which all who have died or "sleep in Christ" will be awakened when Jesus comes to earth the second time (I Thessalonians 4:14-18).   The death that we need to fear is that second death which will start after the second resurrection (Revelation 20:6-15). The second death is hell.

When the scriptures say that the "wages of sin is death" (Romans 6:23), it means that all who have sinned at any time are destined for hell, the second death. The scriptures also say that **ALL** have sinned and fallen short of the glory of God. This means that we all deserve to die in hell. But, thanks to our Lord and Savior, Jesus Christ, the penalty has been paid for our sins.

Jesus, a member of the Godhead, came down from His throne in glory. He walked the earth as a man and suffered every temptation that any human being has had to suffer. Throughout His life on earth, He never sinned once. When His time came, He died on the cross at Calvary. He died to pay the price for our sins.   Jesus suffered extensively for us. He literally took our place in hell and died that "second" death for us. In other words, He went to hell for us and saved us from that awful experience; thus, the title "savior". He shed His precious blood, the ultimate **FOUNTAIN OF YOUTH**, that we may have eternal life. This is the greatest gift that the world has ever received.

> "Greater love hath no man than
> this, that a man lay down his
> life for his friends.
> Ye are my friends, if ye do
> whatsoever I command you."
> John 15:13-14

Without the shedding of blood (Jesus Christ's blood) there is no remission of Sin. We are saved by the precious blood of Jesus Christ.

> "And almost all things are by
> the law purged with blood; and
> without shedding of blood is
> no remission.
> Hebrews 9:22

> "So Christ was once offered to
> bear the sins of many; and
> unto them that look for him
> shall he appear the second time
> without sin unto salvation."
> Hebrews 9:28

Keeping our blood healthy is a key factor in providing us a healthy experience on earth. Being washed in the **BLOOD OF THE LAMB (JESUS CHRIST)** allows us to live forever.

We have one addendum to Leg 14, "What Can We Expect From Following The Health Laws?" Now that we have concluded our study, we know that if we follow all 11 Health Laws (including "The Ultimate Principle of Health: A Personal Relationship With God: Faith, Trust, Obedience, Prayer, Study and Unselfish Service), discussed in Leg 18...,

WE CAN EXPECT

TO LIVE FOREVER ! !

THERE IS A FOUNTAIN

There is a fountain filled with blood, Drawn from Immanuel's veins;
And sinners plunged beneath that flood, Lose all their guilty stains,
Lose all their guilty stains, Lose all their guilty stains;
And sinners plunged beneath that flood, Lose all their guilty stains.

The dying thief rejoiced to see That fountain in his day;
And there may I, though vile as he, Wash all my sins away,
Wash all my sins away, Wash all my sins away;
And there may I, though vile as he, Wash all my sins away.

Thou dying Lamb! Thy precious blood Shall never lose its power,
Till all the ransomed church of God Are saved, to sin no more,
Are saved to sin no more, Are saved to sin no more;
Till all the ransomed church of God Are saved, to sin no more.

E'er since by faith I saw the stream Thy flowing wounds
supply,
Redeeming love has been my theme, And shall be till I
die,
And shall be till I die, And shall be till I die;
Redeeming love has been my theme, And shall be till I
die.

Lord, I believe Thou hast prepared, Unworthy though I
be,
For me a blood-bought, free reward, a golden harp for
me!
A golden harp for me! A golden harp for me!
For me a blood-bought, free reward, a golden harp for
me!

There is a nobler, sweeter song, I'll sing Thy power to
save,
When this poor lisping, stammering tongue Is ransomed
form the grave,
Is ransomed from the grave, Is ransomed from the grave;
When this poor lisping, stammering tongue Is ransomed
from the grave.

William Cowper, 1770 (1731-1800)
Cleansing Fountain C.M.D.
Early American Melody

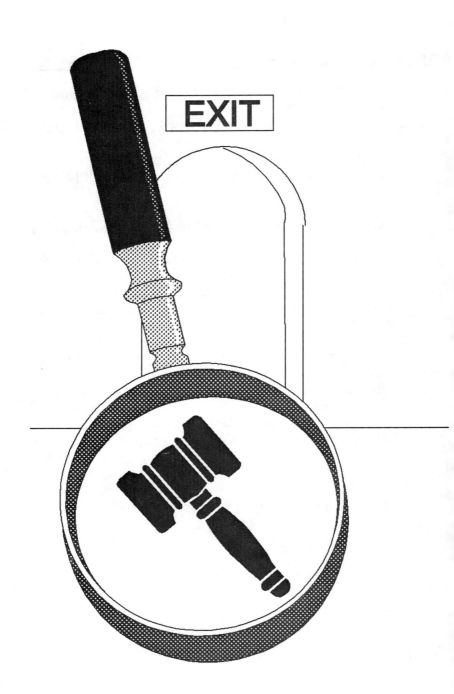

LEG 20

LET US HEAR THE CONCLUSION OF THE WHOLE MATTER:

FEAR GOD, AND KEEP HIS COMMANDMENTS: FOR THIS IS THE WHOLE DUTY OF MAN

W E started on a journey **In SEARCH OF THE FOUNTAIN OF YOUTH** and found it. We learned a lot of glorious information which will not only help us in this life, but even shed light on how we can attain life eternal.

Our soar through **STRESS MANAGEMENT** taught us that life is more complex than just living healthily and waiting to move into eternity. Many things happen to us while we are living on planet earth. Some of them cause great distress; yet, we have no control over some of them, nor do we understand why we must suffer through them.

We are born, we live, we learn, we love, we work, we worry, we gain possessions, we lose possessions, we hurt, we cry, and we reproduce. There are happy times when we accomplish nice things like diplomas, good job promotions, and meet that someone special and get married. There are other times when we study and prepare for a certain job or a promotion for years, only to find that someone else was given the position. Frequently, the person may be less qualified than we are; but, it doesn't matter--they still get the job.

Many people lose loved ones through death or divorce. Sometimes our best friends move away and we never hear from them again. Others go through the pain of living fifty or sixty years with one mate only to lose this person in death at a time when the one left behind is most vulnerable. Sometimes, some of us have to grieve because we lose our children to crime and violent deaths. Then, there are those who lose people in what is considered a totally senseless event.

We go through all kinds of experiences in this tedious journey on planet earth. There are times when we wonder how we made it through it all. At other times we wonder how we could have so miserably failed such a simple test. Sometimes we look at ourselves in the mirror and feel good about our decisions. Later, we may look at something else and say, "What a stupid mistake".

We are all grossly aware of the fact that this world is not fair. Sometimes we feel mistreated for the benefit of someone else. Sometimes someone else is unjustly on the losing end and we are the benefactor. Many are the times that we have cried as we watched a news program or read a paper about the helpless victim of a despicable, unfortunate act at the hands of some pervert.

We go through experience after experience; then, at some point, no matter how happy, or how healthy we are; we die. All of us, who are living right this moment, will die unless Jesus comes back to planet earth before that happens (and we have accepted Him as our Lord and Savior). When we die the first death, contrary to popular belief, we are not marching around heaven praising God or visiting and advising relatives on planet earth. When we die, we rest until the resurrection (Job 7:9; Ecclesiastes 9:5-6,10 Isaiah 38:18 and I Thessalonians 4:13-18).

Though we understand that if we abide in Jesus we will eventually have eternal life; we wonder, "what is the purpose of life and why is there so much suffering?" After all, if Jesus died for us, as pointed out in Leg 19, why do we still have to suffer down here on planet earth? Why would Christ choose to suffer and go through hell for us when He could just as easily have placed us in heaven from the beginning and avoided all of this.

We, like all people, ponder over such things as: the purpose of life, why there is suffering, and why there are so many things that we do not understand. Do we **DARE** begin another search, this time for the purpose of life. We will suffer it to be so.

ONE FINAL SEARCH

When we started our **SEARCH FOR THE FOUNTAIN OF YOUTH,** we learned that we were not the first to do so. As we look at the Holy scriptures, we learn that; as before, we are not the first to search for the meaning and purpose of life. One person who undertook such a search was King Solomon, the son of David. Solomon wrote the Books of Proverbs, Ecclesiastes, and The Song of Solomon. He talked about his search for wisdom and the meaning of life in 977 B. C. He tried to figure out a reason for everything and tells his story in Ecclesiastes. This particular part of the Bible could be considered Solomon's autobiography.

Solomon was one of the richest and most powerful men of his time. Instead of saying "of his time" we could just as easily have said "that the world has ever known." He had everything that one could imagine; yet, he was not satisfied. All of us, at one time or another, have said, "If only I had more of this or more of that, I would be happy or I would then be able to do...", ad infinitum. Well, Solomon had everything that you and I could probably think to name. He had sixty (yes, that's right 60) wives, eighty concubines, and countless virgins available to him. Yet, he was not satisfied. He turned to drink and folly; yet, he was not made happy. He had great works (gardens, houses, vineyards, orchards, trees planted, pools of water) all built or planted for himself; yet, this did not quench his desires. He had silver, gold, men singers, women singers, and musical instruments of all sorts; yet, he continuously sought for something else. He had great possessions and said, "everything mine eyes desired, I kept not from myself" (Ecclesiastes 2:10), but Solomon searched for something more.

Solomon is known as perhaps one of the wisest men who ever lived. Of his great wisdom he said, "wisdom is of more value than foolishness, just as light is better than darkness; for the wise man sees, while a fool is blind. And yet I noticed that there was one thing that happened to the wise and the foolish alike--just as the fool will die, so will I. So of what value is my wisdom?" (The Living Bible Ecclesiastes 2:11-15).

SOLOMON'S CONCLUSION OF THE MATTER

In summary, Solomon had wisdom, wine, women, song, children, a good family background (he was royalty-- the son of a king and a king himself), political power, wealth, fame, and the respect and attention of all of his peers; but he was not satisfied. He repeatedly set forth to satisfy himself, but was unable to do so until he sought the Lord. He summarizes what he learned from his search in these words, "Let us hear the conclusion of the whole matter: Fear God, and keep his commandments: for this is the whole duty of man," (Ecclesiastes 12:13).

OUR CONCLUSION OF THE MATTER

A thorough search of the Holy Scriptures helps us to understand that we are strangely "caught" in the middle of a battle between the forces of "good" and "evil" with the two sides being ruled by one "real" SUPER POWER (God representing good) and a lesser power (the devil representing evil). Planet earth is the battle ground of this great war (Revelation 12:7-12).

The concept of our being "caught in the middle" is thoroughly illustrated in the experiences of Job. Job was a good man. He loved God and was delighted to obey Him (Job 1:1-22).   Job suffered tremendously at the hands of Satan as God allowed him to be tested. He kept the faith and when the test was finished he was delivered. He had more at the end of his life than he did at the beginning (Job 42:12-17).

All things work together for the good of those who love the Lord (Romans 8:28).   So, while we are conveniently placed in the "middle", God, our Creator (through His infinite wisdom and extensive love) has decided to make this a training ground for us to develop our characters through the trials and tribulations being placed upon us by our foe, Satan.

This explanation helps somewhat; but, we still wonder, if God is love, Why does He allow us to suffer and be tested by Satan? "Allow" is a key word because God never causes suffering, but He does allow it.   And, strangely, He allows it because He is **LOVE**. This really sounds strange; but, when we delve deeper into His character, it does make sense. Let us consider that God is

Love, and The Ten Commandments (the transcript of His character) all hang on love (Matthew 22:37-40). When God chose His character, and authored the Ten Commandments to exemplify it, He placed certain restrictions upon Himself. Now, this sounds even more strange. The God of the universe, restricted. The answer: "Yes". He, by His own choice, has restricted Himself in two ways.

■　　The first restriction that God has placed upon Himself is that He must allow all of His subjects freedom of choice. Because He is love, He has no choice but to let all the thinking creatures that He has made, make their own decisions. He will not force us, against our will, to do things that we don't want to do. To a certain degree, He lets us do as we please.

　　　Of course, He intervenes many times. When we are unsure or plan to do foolish things that we don't understand, sometimes He stops us. Many times when we plan to do harm to others, He will intervene to either stop or curtail the hurt or damage that the other person would suffer.

　　　But, when we understand, and then choose self-destruction, our loving and kind God allows it. When Satan chose to disobey God and start the sin cycle, God could not suddenly change His mind about allowing His subjects "freedom of choice" and jump in and force Satan to do that which was right.

■   The second restriction that God has placed upon Himself is the fact that He too must follow His Ten Commandments. When Jesus Christ (a member of the Godhead) travelled the earth, **HE MADE IT PLAIN THAT HE KEPT THE TEN COMMANDMENTS** (see John 15:10). So, no member of the Godhead can lie, steal, profane the Sabbath, or go against any of the commandments (see John 10:35, Titus 1:2 and Hebrews 6:18). Equally true, they cannot break the sixth Commandment, "Thou shalt not Kill".

    Lucifer, an angel created perfectly, turned himself into Satan, the devil (Isaiah 14:12-21), and God will not kill him. Just as God did not suddenly change His mind about giving His subjects free will-- equally true is the fact that once Satan sinned, God did not suddenly decide to: change His own character, rewrite the Ten Commandments (leaving out the sixth one) and kill Satan. And if He won't change His law, we can be assured that He won't break it.

"Now wait just a minute", we say. "God is not going to kill Satan". "Then, surely we are doomed to eternal misery". No, we are not doomed to eternal misery. Eternal life cannot exist outside of the Life giver. Therefore, when Satan or any of his followers choose to disobey God; they choose to die, but they perish at their own hands (see Romans 1:18-2:23 & Psalms 5:10) not at the hands of God.

    There is one important factor that must be considered, when anyone chooses to disobey God, they choose death. Immediately, they may die spiritually but not physically. This is what happened with Adam and Eve. They were tricked by Satan into eating what they believed was forbidden unto them. But they lived on for hundreds of years. Eventually, they died. Satan, too, will eventually die. But, he will continue his evil deeds until he does.

Once Satan decided to disobey God, sin had to run its course. All will see its destruction and it will not rise a second time. If God planned to finally kill Satan, He would not have allowed us to go through all of this suffering. He would have killed him before the whole world was contaminated with sin. The actions and activities of the evil one will eventually lead to hell fire and the total destruction of sin.

We must remember that God has promised to wipe away all tears after this journey is completed (Revelation 21:4). If we live according to God's purpose, we will be blessed to see all of our friends and loved ones again, even those that we lost through death. Of course they will have had to have died in Christ also.

Although, He has not given us all of the information at this time (I Corinthians 13:12), He has left His word to be a light unto our feet and a lamp unto our paths (Psalms 119:105). He will soon return to this earth to rescue his people. We have examples through His word that when He returns, we will participate in either a resurrection or a translation. Enoch and Elijah represent those who will be alive when He comes. These two people were translated. Moses and Jesus Christ, Himself, represent those who died in Christ. They both were resurrected. Also, others were resurrected when Jesus came from the tomb (Matthew 25:50-53).

What are we to do in the meantime as we wait for Jesus' return? We are to watch, pray, and occupy until He comes (Matthew 14:38 and Luke 19:3). God has given us final victory over all things and we will never be tempted beyond that which we can bear (I Corinthians 10:13).

If God intervened and stopped every potential pain or discomfort and always refused to let anyone ever suffer mistreatment, we would never be able to see the devastation of sin. No matter how bad it gets, we can be mindful that it can get worse. Our Bibles tell us that the angels of the Lord are "holding back the winds of strife" (Revelation 7:1).

Satan is the Prince of this world. He initiates all evil but he does not have complete charge. He has been given some power and a certain amount of control for a "short time" (Revelation 12:12). God does protect us from many things, but when we suffer hardships and find that we or those whom we love are mistreated, it can always be attributed to any one or any combination of the following reasons.

- We brought it upon ourselves by making poor or unhealthy choices.

- It is allowed to be a lesson for us or someone else.

- It will strengthen our characters.

- God is allowing us to be tested.

There is a reason for all suffering, but we may not fully understand it until after the second coming of Christ.

We all love to quote Philippians 4:13, "I can do all things through Christ which strengtheneth me." It is good for us to look above this to verses 11 and 12 which read, "Not that I speak in respect of want: for I have learned, in whatsoever state I am, therewith to be content. I know both how to be abased, and I know how to abound: every where and in all things I am instructed both to be full and to be hungry, both to abound and to suffer need." Paul's statement, "I can do all things through Christ which strengtheneth me" was in reference to his ability to be patient and trust God in His great love and wisdom in whatever circumstances he found himself. We must be ever mindful of the fact that the race is not always given to the swift (Ecclesiastes 9:11), and he that endureth to the end shall be saved (Matthew 10:22).

SUMMARY

We looked at the concerns plaguing the American society today, and noticed that the same topics surfaced over and over. Such topics are: *SUBSTANCE ABUSE*, *CRIME*, *TEEN PREGNANCIES*, *POOR HEALTH*, *THE HIGH COSTS OF HEALTH SERVICES*, *OVERWEIGHT*, *STRESS*, *AND SEARCHING FOR METHODS TO INCREASE THE QUALITY AND QUANTITY OF LIFE*. We noted the tremendous amount of confusion that surrounded the factors which really impact health. We noted that sickness had become accepted as the "status quo".

We were not satisfied with the status quo; so, we began a journey IN SEARCH OF THE FOUNTAIN OF YOUTH. We started our search by taking the time to determine exactly what we were searching for. We then looked at fountains, architecture, engineering, technology, science, the status of American health, and the medical field. We totally agree with Solomon, "much study is a weariness of the flesh", (Ecclesiastes 12:12).

Finally, we learned of the location of the FOUNTAIN OF YOUTH in the HOLY BIBLE. We also learned that the Bible is about six thousand years ahead of medical science.

The final conclusion that we have come to is: The Godhead [(THE FATHER, SON, AND THE HOLY SPIRIT) (Romans 1:20)], creator of the heaven and earth, alone, is in charge of this universe. He or (they if you prefer) has designed the universe in a very specific manner, (Genesis 1:1-31). Anyone who chooses to live counter to that design is choosing destruction (Proverbs 1:20-33). God sits high and looks low because heaven is His throne and the earth is His footstool (Isaiah 66:1). Jesus promised that He would come back for us and He will (II Peter 3:9-11).

We need to love, respect, trust, obey, pray, and have faith in God. We need to love our fellowmen and unselfishly minister to the needs of those who require our services.

Without God, we can do nothing. Our responsibility is **not** to try to figure out why everything that happens, happens nor when and how it does. His thoughts are not our thoughts and His ways are not our ways (Isaiah 55:6-9). Our responsibility is to love Him and keep His commandments and all of His statues of health. (Exodus 15:26, John 14:23), as we patiently wait for His return (John 14:1-4). In the words of Solomon, "FEAR GOD, AND KEEP HIS COMMANDMENTS: FOR THIS IS THE WHOLE DUTY OF MAN."

"ALL THIS IS TRUTH", CREATOR OF THE HEAVEN AND THE EARTH.

IN Search *OF*
The Fountain Of Youth

APPENDIX, REFERENCES, & INDEX

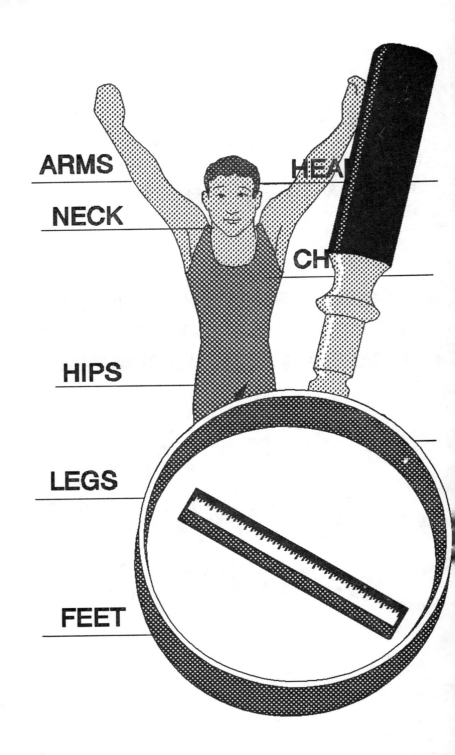

ARMS

HEAD

NECK

CH

HIPS

LEGS

FEET

INITIAL MEASUREMENTS

DATE _____   NAME _____   AGE ____

HEIGHT _____   WEIGHT _____   BLOOD PRESSURE _____

PULSE _____   RESPIRATION _____   HEART RATE _____

CHEST/BREAST _____   WAIST _____

BODY FAT

This section is optional, these measurements are available to you only if you have access to calipers.

WAIST GIRTH _____   % BODY FAT ____

BICEPS _____   TRICEPS _____   SUPRAILIAC _____

ABDOMEN _____

SUBJECTIVE ASSESSMENT

WEIGHT HISTORY

1.   My ideal weight is _____.

2.   I am ____ pounds over/under my ideal weight.

3.   The length of time that I have been overweight is _____.

4.   The length of time that I have been under weight is _____.

5.   My highest adult weight was/is _____. (When) _____.

6.   My lowest adult weight was/is _____. (When) _____.

6.   My weight problem started (when) _____.

7.   The events/problems which were occurring when my weight
      problems started were:

      _____

      _____

      _____

      _____

8.   My patterns of gaining/losing weight are:

      _____

      _____

      _____

      _____

DIET HISTORY

1.   I have attempted reduction diets ____ times.

2.   The average length of time on the diets was ____.

3.   The average number of pounds lost was _____.

EXERCISE HISTORY

1.   I exercise for _____ minutes per session and I have ___ sessions per week.

2.   I have been exercising for _____ weeks/months/years.

HEALTH HABITS ASSESSMENT

Write the number which most closely corresponds to how you really are on the line adjacent to it. Add up all of the numbers and see the rating scale at the end of the assessment.

1.   On the average day I feel
       _____ 5 Great
       _____ 4 Good
       _____ 2 Tired
       _____ 0 Sick

2.   Unless fasting, I eat breakfast
       _____ 5 Daily
       _____ 4 Frequently
       _____ 3 Occasionally
       _____ 2 Rarely
       _____ 0 Never

3.   When I leave the table I feel stuffed
       _____ 0 After each meal
       _____ 1 Frequently
       _____ 3 Occasionally
       _____ 4 Rarely
       _____ 5 Never

4.　　I suffer from indigestion
　　　____　0　Daily
　　　____　1　Frequently
　　　____　3　Occasionally
　　　____　4　Rarely
　　　____　5　Never

5.　　I suffer with constipation
　　　____　0　Daily
　　　____　1　Frequently
　　　____　2　Occasionally
　　　____　4　Rarely
　　　____　5　Never

6.　　I add salt to my food at the table
　　　____　0　Daily
　　　____　1　Frequently
　　　____　2　Occasionally
　　　____　3　Rarely
　　　____　5　Never

7.　　I eat desserts
　　　____　0　Daily
　　　____　1　Frequently
　　　____　2　Occasionally
　　　____　3　Rarely
　　　____　5　Never

8.　　I consume alcohol
　　　____　0　Daily
　　　____　0　Frequently
　　　____　0　Occasionally
　　　____　0　Rarely
　　　____　5　Never

9. When I eat bread it is
    ____ 2 White (enriched)
    ____ 5 Whole grain

10. I drink soft drinks
    ____ 0 Daily
    ____ 0 Frequently
    ____ 3 Occasionally
    ____ 4 Rarely
    ____ 5 Never

11. I drink coffee
    ____ 0 Daily
    ____ 0 Frequently
    ____ 2 Occasionally
    ____ 3 Rarely
    ____ 5 Never

12. I drink tea containing caffeine
    ____ 0 Daily
    ____ 1 Frequently
    ____ 2 Occasionally
    ____ 3 Rarely
    ____ 5 Never

13. I use butter, margarine
    ____ 0 Daily
    ____ 1 Frequently
    ____ 2 Occasionally
    ____ 3 Rarely
    ____ 5 Never

14. I eat ____ meal(s) a day (T.N.T.C. = Too Numerous to Count)
    ____ 0 T.N.T.C.
    ____ 1 Four
    ____ 3 Three
    ____ 5 Two

15. I eat pork _____ times a week
     ____ 0 Daily
     ____ 1 Frequently
     ____ 2 Occasionally
     ____ 3 Rarely
     ____ 5 Never

16. I eat beef _____ times a week
     ____ 0 Daily
     ____ 2 Frequently
     ____ 3 Occasionally
     ____ 4 Rarely
     ____ 5 Never

17. I eat other red meat ____ a week
     ____ 0 Daily
     ____ 2 Frequently
     ____ 3 Occasionally
     ____ 4 Rarely
     ____ 5 Never

18. I catch colds _____
     ____ 0 Frequently   (5-6 per year)
     ____ 1 Occasionally (3-4 per year)
     ____ 3 Rarely   (about once a year)
     ____ 4 very seldom   (less than once a year)
     ____ 5 Never

19. I feel nervous
     ____ 0 Daily
     ____ 1 Frequently
     ____ 3 Occasionally
     ____ 4 Rarely
     ____ 5 Never

20.   I sleep soundly
       ____ 5 Nightly
       ____ 4 Frequently
       ____ 3 Occasionally
       ____ 1 Rarely
       ____ 0 Never

21.   I feel helpless
       ____ 0 Daily
       ____ 1 Frequently
       ____ 3 Occasionally
       ____ 4 Rarely
       ____ 5 Never

22.   I feel depressed
       ____ 0 Daily
       ____ 1 Frequently
       ____ 3 Occasionally
       ____ 4 Rarely
       ____ 5 Never

23.   I am ___ pounds over or under my ideal weight
       ____ 5 Ten   (within 10 or at my ideal weight)
       ____ 4 Fifteen
       ____ 3 Twenty
       ____ 1 Twenty five
       ____ 0 Thirty

24.   I have chest pain
       ____ 0 Daily
       ____ 0 Frequently
       ____ 1 Occasionally
       ____ 3 Rarely
       ____ 5 Never

25.   I smoke
       ____ 0 Daily
       ____ 0 Frequently
       ____ 1 Occasionally
       ____ 3 Rarely
       ____ 5 Never

26.   I take time to relax and enjoy my meals at each mealtime.
       ____ 5 Daily
       ____ 4 Frequently
       ____ 3 Occasionally
       ____ 1 Rarely
       ____ 0 Never

27.   I fast at least
       ____ 5 Weekly
       ____ 5 Monthly
       ____ 3 Four times a year
       ____ 2 twice a year
       ____ 0 Never

28.   I walk or perform some other type of outside activity
       ____ 5 Daily
       ____ 4 Four days a week
       ____ 3 Three days a week
       ____ 2 Two days a week
       ____ 1 Less than once a week

29.   I eat between meal snacks
       ____ 0 Daily
       ____ 1 Frequently
       ____ 3 Occasionally
       ____ 4 Rarely
       ____ 5 Never

30. I drink ice cold drinks
    ____ 0 Daily
    ____ 1 Frequently
    ____ 3 Occasionally
    ____ 4 Rarely
    ____ 5 Never

31. I drink extremely hot drinks
    ____ 0 Daily
    ____ 1 Frequently
    ____ 3 Occasionally
    ____ 4 Rarely
    ____ 5 Never

32. I stay over to finish my regular work
    ____ 0 Daily
    ____ 1 Often but not daily
    ____ 3 At least weekly
    ____ 4 A few times a month
    ____ 5 Almost never

33. I work on a job where my decisions are _____ to the organization
    ____ 5 Mildly Important
    ____ 3 Important
    ____ 0 Critically Important

34. I have at least one friend or family member with whom I can openly discuss my problems
    ____ 5 Anytime
    ____ 4 Frequently
    ____ 3 Sometimes
    ____ 2 Seldom
    ____ 1 Never

35.   I dress for the weather (i.e. scarf, gloves when cold) etc.
        ____ 5 Always
        ____ 4 Frequently
        ____ 3 Sometimes
        ____ 2 Rarely
        ____ 0 Never

36.   I use over-the-counter drugs
        ____ 5 Never
        ____ 4 Rarely
        ____ 3 Sometimes
        ____ 2 Frequently
        ____ 1 Constantly

37.   I do something that I really enjoy
        ____ 5 Daily
        ____ 4 Bi-weekly
        ____ 3 Monthly
        ____ 2 Seldom
        ____ 0 Never

38.   I feel inadequate to handle new situations
        ____ 5 Never
        ____ 4 Seldom
        ____ 3 Sometimes
        ____ 2 Frequently
        ____ 1 Always

39.   I habitually condemn myself for mistakes and shortcomings
        ____ 5 Never
        ____ 4 Seldom
        ____ 3 Sometimes
        ____ 2 Frequently
        ____ 0 Constantly

40.   I have a strong need for approval and recognition by other people
   - _____ 5 Never
   - _____ 4 Seldom
   - _____ 3 sometimes
   - _____ 2 Frequently
   - _____ 0 Constantly

SCORING INFORMATION

Remember, this test is not to be considered as a "scientific" assessment of your health status. It is merely a very simple guideline that can be used to help you see health improvements as you begin to practice the health laws.

RATING SCALE

200 -   Are you sure?

150 - 199   Your health is probably very good.

100 - 149   Your present status of health is probably fair; yet, there is room for improvement.

0 - 99   It is important that you begin making changes immediately.

REFERENCES

Academic American Encyclopedia. Grolier Incorporated, Danburg, Connecticut, Volumes 1-20, 1988.

Anthony, Catherine Parker, & Kolthoff, Norma Jane. *Textbook of Anatomy and Physiology,* Ninth Edition, The C. V. Mosby Company, Saint Louis, 1975

Austin, Phyllis; Thrash, Agatha; & Thrash, Calvin. *More Natural Remedies,* Thrash Publications, Seale, Alabama.

Blotchy, Mark J.; Grace, Keith; & Looney, John G. "CLINICAL EXPERIENCE Treatment of Adolescents in Family Therapy after Divorce", *Journal of the American Academy if Child Psychiatry,* 23, 2:222-225, 1984.

Bullough, Bonnie & Bullough, Vern L. *The Emergence of Modern Nursing,* The Macmillan Company, New York, Collier-Macmillan Limited, London, 1966.

Cagney, J. Kenneth. *Beating Drug & Alcohol Problems in the Workplace: Detection, Control & Treatment,* Business and Legal Reports Bureau of Law and Business. Inc. Hazardous Waste Bulletin 64 Wall Street, Madison, 1986.

Cassell, Eric J. & Siegler, Mark. *Changing Values in Medicine* (Papers delivered at the Conference on Changing Values in Medicine, Cornell University Medical College, New York City, November 11-13, 1979), University Publications of America, Inc.

Castiglioni, Arturo. *A History of Medicine,* (Translated from the Italian and Edited by E. B. Krumbhaar), Second Edition, Published simultaneously in Canada by The Ryerston Press manufactured in the United States, 1947.

Clinical Pediatrics, June 1983, p. 449, (Clinical Note), "Alcohol-related Highway Fatalities Among Young Drivers".

Clute, Michael F. *Into the Father's Heart: A Shocking Revelation,* God's Last Call Ministries, Newberg, Oregon, 1982.

Clute, Michael F. *The Wonderful Truth About Our Heavenly Father,* God's Last Call Ministries, Newberg, Oregon, 1985.

Collier's Encyclopedia, Macmillian Educational Company, New York, P. F. Collier, Inc. London & New York 1987, Volumes 1-23.

Compton's Encyclopedia and Fact Index, Compton's Learning Company, A Division of Encyclopaedia Britannica. Inc. Chicago, 1989, Volumes 1-25.

De Jong, Allan R. "The Medical Evaluation of Sexual Abuse in Children", *Hospital and Community Psychiatry,* May 1985, Vol. 36, No. 5

Dixon, Richard, E. "Nosocomial Infection: A Continuing Problem" *Postgraduate Medicine,* Vol. 62. No. 2, August 1977.

Dock, Lavinia L. & Stewart, Isabel M. *A Short History of Nursing,* G. P. Putnam's sons, New York : London, 1938.

Dolan, Josephine A. *Goodnow's HISTORY OF NURSING,* W. B. Saunders Company, Philadelphia & London, 1964.

The EarthWorks Group. *50 Simple Things You Can Do To Save The Earth,* Earthworks Press; Berkeley, California; 1989.

Edlin, Gordon & Golanty, Eric. *HEALTH & WELLNESS A Holistic Approach,* Jones and Bartlett Publishers, Boston Portola Valley, 1988.

The Encyclopedia American International Edition, Grolier Incorporated, International Headquarters: Danbury, Connecticut Volumes 1-29, 1987.

Encyclopedia International, Lexicon Publications, Inc. Volumes 1-19, 1981.

Garrison, Fielding H. *Contributions to The History of Medicine* from the Bulletin of the New York Academy of Medicine 1925-1935, Hafner Publishing Company, Inc. New York, London, 1966.

Gomes-Schwartz, Beverly; Horowitz, Jonathan M.; & Sauzier, Maria. "Severity of Emotional Distress Among Sexual Abused Preschool, School-Age and Adolescent Children", *Hospital and Community Psychiatry,* May 1985, Vol. 36, No. 5.

Gorton, David Allyn. *The History of Medicine,* Philosophical and Critical, from Its Origin to the Twentieth Century, G. P. Putnam's Sons, New York and London, 1910.

Gray's Anatomy, Thirty-Seventh Edition, (Edited by Peter L. Williams, Roger Warwick, Mary Dyson & Lawrence H. Bannister, Churchill Livingstone, Edinburgh London Melbourne and New York, 1989.

Green, Wayne, H.; Campbell, Magda; & David, Raphael. "Psychosocial Dwarfism: A Critical Review of the Evidence", *Journal of the American Academy of Child Psychiatry*, 23, 1:39-48, 1984.

The HOLY BIBLE, King James Version (unless otherwise indicated).

Jacob, Stanley W. & Francone, Clarice Ashworth. *Structure and Function in Man*, Third Edition, W. B. Saunders Company, Philadelphia, London & Toronto, 1974.

Jensen, Deborah Maclurg. *History and Trends of Professional Nursing*, Third Edition, The C. V. Mosby Company, St. Louis, 1955.

Johnson, Jerry A. *WELLNESS: A Concept for Living*, SLACK Inc. Thorofare, New Jersey, 1986.

Hoffman, Milton Jay. *HUNZA: Fifteen Secrets of the Healthiest and Oldest Living People*, Professional Press Publishing Association, Valley Center, California, 1979.

THE HUMANITY OF THE ILL: Phenomenological Perspectives, Edited by Victor Kestenbaum, The University of Tennessee Press, Knoxville, 1982.

"Improving Health Care Through Research and Development", Report of the Panel on Health Services Research Development of the President's Science Advisory Committee; Office of Science and Technology Executive Office of the President, March 1972.

Kaplan, Stuart L.; Landa, Beth; Weinhold, Chantel; & Shenker, Ronald I. "Adverse Health Behaviors and Depressive Symptomatology in Adolescents", *Journal of the American Academy of Child Psychiatry,* 23, 595-601, 1984.

Kloss, Jethro. *BACK TO EDEN,* A Human Interest Story of Health and Restoration To Be Found in Herb, Root, and Bark (Revised and Expanded Second Edition), Back to Eden Books Publishing Co., 1988.

Lederman, E. K. *Philosophy and Medicine,* Revised Edition, Gower Publishing Company, Vermont, 1986.

Life & Health: National Health Journal, VEGETARIANISM, Review and Herald Publishing Association, Vol. 1 Second Edition, Washington, D.C., 1973.

The Life Management Group. *"The Blue Cross & Blue Shield Guide to Staying Well",* Contemporary Books, Inc. Chicago, 1982.

Mann, George V. "Saccharin--Sweet and Dangerous", *Postgraduate Medicine,* Vol. 62, No. 1, July 1977.

Mettler, Cecilia C. & Mettler, Fred A. *History of Medicine,* The Blakiston Company, Philadelphia, Toronto, 1947.

National Data Book and Guide to Sources STATISTICAL ABSTRACT OF THE UNITED STATES 1988, 108th Edition, U.S. Department of Commerce, C. William Verity, Secretary & Robert Ortner, Under Secretary for Economic Affairs. Bureau of the Census John G. Keane, Director. December 1987.

The New Encyclopaedia Britannica, Encyclopaedia Britannica, Inc. Volumes 1-12, Chicago, 1990.

Null, Gary & Steve. *The Complete Handbook of Nutrition,* Dell Publishing Company, New York, New York, 1981.

Nutting, Adelaide M. & Dock, Lavinia L. *A History of Nursing,* G. P. Putnam's Sons, New York and London, 1935.

Physicians' Desk Reference, Forty-third Edition, Medical Economics Company Inc., Oradell, N. J., 1989.

Podell, Richard N. (Nutrition Highlights) "Food, Mind, and Mood: Hyperactivity Revisited", *Hyperactivity,* Vol. 78/NO August Post- Graduate Medicine, 1985.

Purtilo, David T. "Diet, Nutrition, and Cancer: An Update of a Controversial Relationship", *Postgraduate Medicine,* Vol. 78/No. 1/July 1985.

Reeder, Sharon, J.; Mastroianni Jr., Luigi; Martin, Leonide L. *Maternity Nursing,* 15th Edition, J. B. Lippincott Company, Philadelphia, 1983.

Robinson, D. E. *The Story of our Health Message,* Third Edition, Southern Publishing Company; Nashville, Tennessee, 1965.

Salzinger, Suzanne; Kaplan, Sandra; Pelcovitz, David; Samit, Carol; & Krieger, Renee. *Journal of the American Academy of Child Psychiatry,* 23, 4:458-464, 1984.

Schultz, Myron G. "Exotic Diseases: Ounce of Prevention or Pound of Cure?" *Postgraduate Medicine,*

Selye, Hans, *The Stress of Life,* Revised Edition, McGraw-Hill Book Co., New York, 1976.

Shelp, Earl E. *Justice and Health Care,* D. Reidel Publishing Company, Dordrecht : Holland / Boston : U.S.A. London : England, 1981.

Siegel, Alberta E. (EDITORIAL) 'Working Mothers and Their Children", *Journal of the American Academy of Child Psychiatry,* p. 486-488, 1984.

Singer, Charles & Underwood, Ashworth E. *A Short History of Medicine,* Second Edition, Oxford University Press, New York & Oxford, 1962.

Skryock, Richard H. *THE HISTORY of NURSING An Interpretation of the Social and Medical Factors Involved,* W. B. Saunders Company, Philadelphia & London, 1959.

Swift, William J., & Letven, Ronelle (Clinical Experience) "Bulemia and the Basic Fault: A Psychoanalytic Interpretation of the Binging-Vomiting Syndrome", *Journal of the American Academy of Child Psychiatry,* 23, 4, 489-497, 1984.

Thrash, Agatha, & Thrash, Calvin. *HOME REMEDIES: Hydrotherapy, Message, Charcoal, and Other Simple Treatments* Thrash Publications, Yuchi Pines Institution; Seale, Alabama, 1981.

Thrash, Agatha, & Thrash, Calvin. *Nutrition For Vegetarians,* Thrash Publications, Yuchi Pines Institution; Seale, Alabama, 1982.

Volkmar, Fred R.; Poll, Joan; & Lewis, Melvin. Conversion Reactions in Childhood and Adolescence, *Journal of the American Academy of Child Psychiatry,* 23, 4:424-430, 1984.

Walker, N. J. *Raw Vegetable Juices,* Jove Publications Inc. New York, (Berkley Publishing Group), 1989.

Weathersbee, Paul S.; Olsen, Larry K.; & Lodge, Robert. (Topics in Primary Care) "Caffeine and Pregnancy" *Postgraduate Medicine,* Vol. 62, No. 3 September 1977.

Welling, Peter. "How Food and Fluid Affect Drug Absorption: Results of Initial Studies", *Postgraduate Medicine* Vol. 62 No. 1 July 1977.

White, Ellen G. *Counsels on Diet and Foods,* Review and Herald Publishing Association, Takoma Park, Washington, D.C., 1976.

White, Ellen G. *Education,* Pacific Press Publishing Association, Mountain View, California; Oshawa, Ontario, 1952.

White, Helene Raskin; Johnson, Valerie; & Horwitz, Allan. An "Application of Three Deviance Theories to Adolescent Substance Use". *The International Journal of the Addictions,* 21(3), 347-366, 1986.

Williams, Peter L.; Warwick, Roger; Dyson, Mary; Bannister, Lawrence H. *Gray's Anatomy* Thirty-Seventh Edition, Churchill Livingston, 1989.

The World Book Encyclopedia, World Book, Inc. A Scott Fetzer Company. Chicago, Volumes 1-21, 1991.

INDEX

"My Work Must Be **DONE, COMPLETED** and **FINISHED**." Our LORD and SAVIOR, Jesus Christ, Creator of the Heaven and Earth.